EAT BUTTER
SMOKE MARIJUANA
KILL CANCER and
LIVE TO 100 YEARS OLD!

Alvin Jackson
"The Most Passionate Non-Doctor On The Internet"

HumanHealthLink.com

Copyright © 2017

Dedication

To my beautiful *wife*, I love hearing about your day and feeling your hugs around my neck while I worked hard on this book. Thank you for being there when I needed you most. Thanks to my kids as well for your loving support.

To my *Dad and Mom*, who talked to me on the phone every Friday or Saturday night to let me know what was happening with the family. Even more than that, you all encouraged me to go for more in life.

I love you, seriously...Thank you.

To my *little brother* who is always striving for more, you'll get it because you just won't quit! I love you Lil' Brother.

One more person I'd like to personally thank **Bryan Sparkman** for his powerful words that kept me on my grind in the writing of this book.

Well...just a few more people. Special thanks go out to all **my students** for their many suggestions and show ideas. I can't thank you all enough for your comments and family stories.

Your Personal Message from Alvin J.

Thank you for picking up this book when there are so many options out there for you to choose from. My gratitude for you spending your time watching me online and picking up this informational health guide is overflowing!

Let's get right into it...I can't stomach the way our government, in line with corrupt corporations, continue to take away our constitutional rights and directly poison our food supply. That's not OK with me! Drugs are pushed onto the market within 2 WEEKS without any consideration for safety, testing, or human regard! Where is our FDA? Oh, yeah. Taking money to allow this nefarious activity continue. Wake up! It's a kick in the gut for every citizen of this country and it has to stop. This is my contribution to help stem this global pandemic of death!

Having said that, YOU now have information in your hands to slow, stop, and totally reverse most diseases that prevail today. Listen, if you buy this book, read it, and use the "gold" encased in these chapters, you can obliterate almost any medical condition known to man, including STAGE 4 CANCERS. On the flip side, if you bought this powerful literature, took the time to read it, then put NOTHING into practice, YOU are right in the same boat as the murderous scum who'd rather see us die than successfully thrive! YOU are enemy #1. You are a danger onto yourself. The most read book in human history said, "...faith without works is dead." I have faith YOU will follow through and save yourself from this tyrannical system.

MY IMMEASURABLE VISION: My fellow human being, there is no other more pressing dilemma to me than the present and future wellbeing of YOU. Without a bunch of "YOUs", there is no us, and without us, there is no world as we know it. We are free as humans to "kick off" this planet anytime we want. Some of us want to end our existence and move on the next Ether. Others of us want to hang around and see what more this life can surprise us with. No matter which one you choose, no other human has the right to deprive another of the right to choose their ending! Someone has to give a damn about YOU...and that someone is ME. □

Content Guide

Disclaimer for Alvin Jackson and Human Health Link:

I am NOT a doctor, nor do I give medical advice. All information put forth in this book and on the Human Health Link website are for entertainment purposes only. No information in this book or on the Human Health Link website is meant to cure, treat, or diagnose any disease, syndrome, disorder, or condition at any time for any reason. No surgeries have been, are, or will be performed in the course of delivering this information. No statements given have been evaluated by the Food and Drug Administration.

No results are guaranteed or implied from the case studies presented. The case study participants have agreed to give their successful accounts of their own free will and were not compensated for their participation. Their outcomes may not be yours, as these participants have followed the directions given closely and consistently over time to gain the results obtained.

Now that we are done with that, let's move on...

Case Study (unedited):

Message Body: Hello, Alvin Jackson ~ Here is my comment of your positive videos of Natural Health care...First I would like to share a portion of my medical background since 1962 ,the purpose of this is to reveal to you how fortunate to find you on youtube. 1962 was diagnosed of a bone cancer,was 2 years old that year. Surgery was performed 3 times in removal of the cancer on right jaw bone & 1 inch from my brain. Was said that I may die in 4 months.... Was said after the 4 months that if I made it to 10 years of age that I would be free of cancer. >>>Got to admit that MD's certainly are not prophets,most of all unnatural healers! Had Many treatments through out childhood,starting from 1969 several reconstructive surgeries were performed to my upper teens. Want to add that Doctors were well trusted in as well as a hospital for many years that I had considdered this enviroment a home, away from home. Until about 5 years ago I had discovered over and over the facts of doctors and pill happy get rich NON health care professionals. I have complained about the above issue,it hit me like a big slap in the face!!!! They are the ones who should be jailed and given their own medicine,chemicals,making them the Biggest drug pushers Ever, not to mention that I have to take drugs for Eppilepsy since a kid. Alvin there is soooo much I could add of negative results from doctors,am glad to see there are Natural doctors speaking out against the MD's!!!! .... ((My comment after finding your videos, and dam I feel GOOD listening to you speak of what is Natural Health and anyone who pays attention will benifit)) ..Yes,your humor is an extra with your presentations. Two main videos below that have been of support and increased my awareness. 1. 30 days to end Diabetees ... This video really motivated me to consume more healther foods which I am doing my best with what I can afford. Feeling more energetic as this body stand a better chance to heal itself,naturally. Threw out diabetic dope 3 or 4 years ago,knew something was wrong taking the drugs presented by doctor > PILL. 2. Get rid of your glasses fast ... The two exercises you presented are very helpful...Because of cancer several years ago left me able to see with only one eye,with love to do the one with the sun but not able in my area ....,I trust I will soon because vision has been fading. Being aware of your messages is the first step and more than glad that someone like yourself is sharing valuable knowledge. Hope others step up to the plate also and walk over the bull shit of using drugs to cover the symptoms, rather than looking for the CAUSE! Looking foward to your youtube channel for more Good info. ... Thank you for your effort to help others from your Heart ~ Earnest / Namaste ~

A Story

Naturopaths vs. Doctors

Let food be thy medicine, and Medicine be thy food.

-Hippocrates

Hey everybody this is Alvin J, the most passionate non-doctor on the internet. Today we talk about how we got into this sticky mess that we now call a "health care system", which is more of a disease management system. Now, don't get me wrong. I believe that the healthcare system is necessary but only for emergencies!

I love movies, so I'll started off this way...Movies often start with us right in the middle of an action scene and that is where I want to take you today. We actually look at the healthcare system today and believe that it was always like that. However, I know for a fact that it is nowhere near where it started and we are light years away from where it should be!

Here's a story that's really not a story at all...

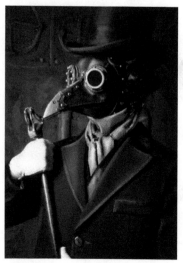

The photo on your left is the photo of a doctor. Strange, isn't it? This was the normal uniform of a doctor in the 17th century. The uniform was invented by a man named Charles de L'orme in 1619 to protect doctors from the plague during that time. Creepy!

The nose of the mask was often stuffed with fragrant herbs to prevent the doctors from breathing in microorganisms. The mask was also meant to protect the eyes of the doctor so that he could see what he was doing. In addition to the mask, there was also a body-length cloth suit that covered the doctor's entire body so no part of his body would be exposed to the plague. As seen in the picture, physicians often poked at the patient with a cane to avoid contact with them all together.

To me, this looks like the ring leader at the Freak Show! These doctors had an interesting repertoire of medieval remedies like draining the blood from your body to cure sickness (blood-letting)! That one also cures LIFE! *LOL* Don't like that, how about having a hole drilled into your skull by a crank drill in order to relieve a headache! No? These are the types of remedies that were offered in the medieval times, and as you can see, they didn't know any better. However, this was considered solid science at the time.

At the exact same time that doctors were delivering these types of "services", there was another group of medical professionals called naturopaths. These professionals were actually known as doctors. Naturopaths felt that human beings had everything within their own bodies to heal. All they needed were fresh grown foods, to keep the patient clean along with rest, and everything else would take care of itself. Indeed, they were right.

Patients chose naturopathic medicine over traditional medicine. So much so that traditional medicine began to fade into non-existence. It doesn't take a genius to see why. When you have a choice of eating fresh, organic vegetables to get yourself well or having a hole drilled into your cranium, there's not much of a choice there!

Enter the Rockefellers. John D. Rockefeller wanted to conquer an industry that would bring him great wealth, thus, he set his sights on the medical industry. One of Rockefeller's most famous sayings was that "competition is a sin". John decided to destroy all competition in opposition to traditional Western medicine. John hired a man named Abraham Flexner to submit a special report to Congress in 1910, basically informing all of Congress that anything outside of Western traditional medicine would be known as "quackery" and severely ineffective.

With John D. Rockefeller's enormous wealth and influence, the plot worked. Because the message came directly from Congress, people believed that fruits and vegetables along with rest could not possibly do what surgeries, pills, and radiation could do. This began the age of corruption in medicine and added to Rockefeller's already enormous fortune.

Fast-forward to today...

How do we look at doctors today? They are the pinnacle of medical intelligence. We trust doctors with our deepest, darkest, most embarrassing secrets. Our doctors know what diseases we have, they've seen us naked, and they even know (sometimes) whether we will live or die!

The media portrays them as heroes. We see them performing miraculous surgeries on patients and bringing them back to full health! Our doctors are often involved in tedious research that took years or even decades to complete. On the news, they even claim to have a cure for cancer. All of these positive accolades that are laid on doctors and make us believe they are competent, supremely intelligent, and ultimately trustworthy. Ah, the media. How it all has changed.

The real media that we *had* in this country used to be annoyingly inquisitive, unrelenting, and downright demanding! That seems to have all gone away nowadays, seeing as how pharmaceutical companies, banks, and large corporations now own all of the media outlets. At present, Rupert Murdoch can easily manipulate the message of his media empire to sway the beliefs of the average, non-inquiring American. Also, Jeff Bezos, the founder of Amazon.com, is the sole owner of the Washington Post. Talk about a conflict of interest!

Now our media swears up and down that doctors are the end-all-be-all of the medical world. I found the doctors are an exact representation of the society that we live in. If you haven't read any statistics lately, most of the people in any society around the world are average or below average at best. If you are reading this book, you are on the above average side. Our doctors come from the same pool of mediocrity as our inept politicians and look how well that turned out.

One other thing you should be acutely aware of is doctors, surgeons, and general health practitioners are all a protected monopoly. This means if your grandmother dies, if you are sister dies, or if your dad dies on the operating table, there is no recourse for you and no punishable law for that doctor.

Let me be clear, there are always good doctors in the world doing their best to make sure that our health is at the forefront of whatever treatments or procedures that they prescribe. If you happen to break a leg, have an appendix rupture, or have an acute aneurysm, I WANT you to go to the emergency room of your nearest hospital. However, if you are in the doctor's office, hospital, or clinic every single day looking for drugs or help from medical professionals, I have it on good authority your life will end prematurely!

Let's talk about the meaning of the title of this book. In the coming chapters, you will learn the benefits of butter, weed, and other things you had no idea would endow you with a healthy lifestyle. Let's get to it!

Section One

Butter, Marijuana, and Killing Cancer

Secret #1: Basting Yourself

Haha! I know, I know. Some of you are thinking "what the hell is Alvin J. doing talking about butter and good health in the same sentence?" Right? Well that's none of your business! I'm just kidding, that's the reason you bought this book. So of course, I'm going to tell you. *LOL*

Now seriously, if I we're talking about Country Crock spread or if I were talking about Imperial Margarine, then you'd have a real reason to be concerned. To be brutally honest with you, those are nothing but free radicals floating around in a bucket waiting to give you cancer. I don't say these words lightly. So please don't take this as me trying to steer you away from some of your favorite, delectable treats.

There are millions of people who are having severe autoimmune diseases, congestive heart failure, and acute brain damage. In my personal opinion, I think these are the reasons for some of the things happening to us health-wise in the United States. If you combine that with childhood vaccinations, a diet stricken with chemicals and preservatives, electromagnetic fields from our phones, chemtrails in the air every day, and the industrial dyes that are cooked into our soaps, toothpaste, and bed sheets, you would see that we have a pretty amazing pandemic of death going on right now!

Having said all that, let's talk about the good butter, the butter that you can actually eat that will cause your body to work properly like we want it to. Anytime we eat butter, it's supposed to be 100% pure butter. If you are eating anything else besides 100% pure butter, you are inundating your body with cancer-causing glop!

I can hear some of you asking the question right now in your head: I've been told all my life that butter is bad for us, so how can we eat butter every day and still remain healthy? Did I hit your question on the head? Being that this is a completely fair question, let me give you the answer.

We were told a lot of things in the early days that didn't make sense for us then that makes total sense now. Remember when you learned in science class that the Earth was round? However, when you actually walked on the surface of this big ole blue ball it appears flat because the surface is so massive. In fact, there is a Flat Earth Society that actually hold meetings and discusses how they will not fall off the edge of the Earth! That is no bullsh**! They actually do exist.

At one time, we also believed (as I mentioned earlier) that drilling a hole into the side of your head would actually let the bad spirits out to rid you of your headache! These are beliefs we no longer hold; thus, you should be able to grasp this concept pretty easily. Butter is our friend, not the enemy! I don't want you going to the grocery store and tiptoeing down the aisle afraid to look at real butter for fear that your health will get worse for eating it.

The truth is...YOU NEED IT! Believe me, I understand. You've gone to your doctor and they've told you that butter is the devil! Well, I'm going to tell you that butter is one of the most amazing and effective foods that we can eat to improve our health. We must realize that butter contains something that we all need and should be eating on a regular basis. I know what you're thinking, you think it's fat. Right? No, not at all.

The most important ingredient in 100% butter is cholesterol. Yes, that's right, CHOLESTEROL! Wait, wait, wait. You're telling me that the very thing that my doctor says that I should control and stay away from in my diet is one of the most important things in my body?! YES...and that goes double for you ladies.

I can hear another question rattling around in your head: why is cholesterol so important for women? All of you women should know right now that your body is regulated by hormones. Some of you actually hate those hormones because of the astounding number of medical issues they cause within your body. Tell me I'm wrong...you hate it! Imbalance of hormones within a female's body actually causes headaches, backaches, abdominal cramps, endometriosis, PCOS, increase degradation of muscle due to stress, and a host of other debilitating conditions which only the female body deals with.

Now over and above that for females, the men are not free and clear themselves. Cholesterol is necessary for men as well. Men have one major basic hormone within our bodies that actually regulate certain processes and conditions, and that is testosterone. A low testosterone count in a man actually results in narrower shoulders, lowered muscle tone, lighter voice, and an inability to gain powerful erections. If that's not enough to get you to eating butter, I think you have problems! *LOL*

Here's the chaser, cholesterol is the main precursor within our bodies in which we derive most of our hormones. In addition to that, we also build our neurotransmitters from cholesterol. This means we cannot carry out brain functions without a proper amount of cholesterol floating through your system. Without cholesterol, we cannot produce some of the major hormones that we require inside of our body like cortisol. Did I mention cholesterol provides the myelin sheath around our neurons? It does.

Cortisol, the stress hormone, is the most powerful anti-inflammatory known to man! Cortisol is extremely powerful, yet it is only available in short supply. Once we run out of this all-important hormone, our bodies will find other ways to construct it, I.E. stealing precursors from your thyroid gland that actually result in low thyroid production, otherwise known as hypothyroidism. There goes your New Year's resolution for losing weight.

To end this off, I want to clarify. When you need healthy fat, you should be eating avocados, nuts, lentils, and fish oils. Those are what we call healthy

Omega-3 fats. Keep reading, these healthy fats have to be balanced with bad fats in order for our bodies to operate at optimum. So, when you eat an avocado, you should also (in very slight amounts) eat some bacon or chicken that has fat. Yes, I just told you that! My goal is not to turn you into a wheatgrass-sweater-knitting, professional-juice-making, Oaktree-kissing hippie in the mountains of Utah.

My goal IS to turn you into a discerning, label-reading, question-everything leader who takes control of their own health! As Bob Proctor said, "don't be an extra in your own movie". We only have one life here to live, and no one is going to live it for us...especially our government. In fact, if you let the outside world dictate what you do, what you eat, or what you say, then what the f**k are you here for!

Ok, I'm calm now. Whew...

Eat 100% pure butter. Next chapter.

Section One

Butter, Marijuana, and Killing Cancer

Secret #2: Take A Hit Of The Ganja

If you all watched any 1990's movies with a reference to marijuana, you know it's called "the ganja"! No, this is not a Jamaican word. It's actually Sanskrit for hemp. We discovered this magical herb centuries ago and realized the powers it has for healing. As you all know, whenever something naturally heals the body and is very effective, our government has a tendency to step in and stomp all over it! Thanks Mr. Rockefeller. (Heavy sarcasm)

Don't worry, I'm not going to give you some long history lesson about marijuana. I'm going to point out some of the more interesting points of this herb and then tell you how we can apply it in order for it to save your life. I know, I know. Some of you don't need your life saved. However, I feel it's my job to give the best information for the worst-case scenario, then it'll automatically work out for those of you who are not in that bad of a health situation.

I think we all know what's special about marijuana. Sometimes we get a funny, giddy feeling of not having a care in the world. At other times, it's a severe stress reliever! Yet at other times, it's just a substance pushed on to you by your friends in the form of peer pressure to help you fit into an awkward, pot-smoking Friday night.

You might have also heard of another useful substance that is contained within marijuana: THC. Tetrahydrocannabinol is a substance found within marijuana that is actually one of the best-known fighters of any type of cancer within the human body. Here's the kicker, THC will actually attack cancer cells and destroy them without harming any healthy tissues in the body! Now that's what I call effective medical treatment.

Wait, wait, stop! Some of you just got way too excited. Just because marijuana has an overwhelming health benefit, that does not mean that you should go out and harass the Dope man on your local corner for a dime bag!

The reason I don't condone *smoking* of marijuana is because it has 5X the potency of a cigarette. Meaning it will damage your lungs 5X as fast! Not the response you were looking for, I'm sure. Notice, I did not say it would cause lung cancer, just lung damage. Luckily, we don't have to be confined to just *smoking* marijuana. Some of you know all too well that marijuana is now manufactured in a myriad of ways. Case in point, we can get cannabis brownies, candy, cookies, even gummy bears! Yes. Don't you eat that whole gummy bear...you're asking for trouble. Seriously. Take a look...

Let's get something straightened out right now, you can overdose on water! Don't go putting evil thoughts in your head about marijuana and thinking that it's an evil drug and just because the government has classified it as a Class 2 narcotic, that it's dangerous and will kill you. That is not the case at all! If you drink 8 gallons of water in one entire day, at the end of that day, you will die! You don't see water listed as a Class 2 narcotic that will kill the average human, do you?

I don't want anything erroneous to happen to any of you. Therefore, I'd appreciate if you took these guidelines seriously and be especially careful about the amounts of THC consumed through these marijuana edibles. As you can see from the stories I've embedded above, there can be dangerous consequences to overdosing on THC, not particularly marijuana. After all, I have seen friends of mine actually smoke an entire forest of marijuana within a week and have absolutely nothing happen! Don't take too much solace in that, I haven't seen these people since college and they might have gone down a terrible path of deteriorating health after that.

The real hero in all of this is something called cannabis oil. Cannabis oil actually has no negative side effects and kills cancer at the same time. Cannabis oil is often used for late-stage cancers in order to curb some of the detrimental side effects that come along with having these devastating cancers. It gives the patient their appetite back, it helps to calm tremors, and it even helps with diarrhea. I currently reside in a state where marijuana was made legal this year: 2017. Being that governments often have their own agenda, I don't know if cannabis oil will then be considered legal. Marijuana is legal. However, I don't know if cannabis oil will be considered legal even though the oil comes from the leaves of the marijuana plant. Currently, cannabis oil is not legal.

Let's get to some other rather scintillating details about the "dubbage". Have you ever wondered how marijuana is able to help with glaucoma? Well, here's the lowdown. Marijuana actually has a double effect. Marijuana actually contains caffeine which is a **diuretic**. This means your body will excrete extra fluids from the tissues of your body in order to rid yourself of toxins. In addition to this, it's also a **drying agent**. Any swollen tissues inside our bodies will have the additional fluids drained via the use of marijuana. So, the answer is YES! It helps with body-wide swelling.

I'd advocate you all looking around YouTube (Youtube.com) to see real videos of people who are using cannabis oil and other marijuana products to actually cure their fatal cancers. Don't take my word for it. Do your own research!

Let's get you more information in the next chapter.

Section One

Butter, Marijuana, and Killing Cancer

Secret #3: Killing Cancer and Living Beyond 100 Years

Case Study (unedited):

> I have grown up to think that diabetes is a meant to be illness in my family for my father passed away because of that..Though for me i have been in early stages because i just started staying alone and had stopped eating the healthy food which my mom used to prepare because you know how it is its hard for someone like me to cook when im busy everyday as a software developer. i always had a mentality of-which i know saved me not to confront any doctor or take any pill of any kind.. if i'm sick it has to wear off with natural remedies but when i discovered that i can clear off any sickness from my system through alvin jackson's youtube video i got happy and angry at the same time... happy that its all done and angry that the doctors had a hand on the passing of my father for they knew how he could be cured but only thought of their pockets and the system in mind... i thank you alvin for directing me the right way which only 20% of people in this world i think only know of. Thanking you for touching my life for no price....its just like how

One of the best TV series I've ever watched in my life is called 'Breaking Bad'. The baseline of the show is a chemistry teacher named Walter White, who is slowly dying of inoperable lung cancer. Walter makes a life altering decision to take care of his family after his death, but not with a normal retirement. Walter decides to become a meth dealer, actually partnering with a meth addict named Jesse Pinkman. Crazy sh**, huh? If you've never watched it, I won't spoil the ending for you. However, the important point for me here is that Walter had cancer. Mr. White was told that his cancer was terminal, which is why he had little apprehension about manufacturing large amounts of meth, an extremely dangerous undertaking.

The 'Breaking Bad' series lasted from 2008 to 2013. As you can see, these are relatively recent dates for this TV series. I say that to say this, there are important pioneers in the history of fighting cancer who actually discovered truly effective ways of killing cancer as early as the 1920s. This means today, terminal cancer should be a far-gone notion!

I'll mention these men and women in depth later in the following chapters. I just want you to know right now, that cancer has been cured over and over again in the early part of this century. Yet there are still interests that insist cut (surgery), burn (radiation), and poison (chemotherapy) are the best ways of dealing with cancer.

Let me ask you a serious question, what do you believe causes cancer? Some people think that cancer is inevitable. My friends believe cancer just pops up one day and we have to "deal with it". Some people believe that cancer comes on as a result of eating contaminated foods. Still other people believe that cancers are a product of Wrath, for the religious! Now, I'm not sure about that last one, but in the days we're living in now, the aforementioned causes are correct. So...does this have to be true for you?

The latest stats say 2 in 3 people on Earth will have some form of cancer throughout their life. That's 66%! That's very scary when there are 7 billion people on the planet, which means 4.63 billion people will have some form of cancer. I don't want to scare you, but look around the room you're sitting in. Most of the people who are afflicted with cancer will be your family members, your friends, or the people that you work with. This is a scary proposition for any human being to face.

I asked you a minute ago, what do you think causes cancer. Well, what I have found is quite shocking to me. It amazes me that there are so few people willing to take part in their own good health. What causes cancer in our society are the same things that make money in our society. Here are the topical causes I found that have erupted deadly cancers up on our society...

1. **Electromagnetic Fields** - Sources: Computers, tablets, smartphones, gaming systems, microwave ovens, smart TVs, smart refrigerators, smart thermostats, and a host of other small, household electronics.

2. **Modern Food** - Sources: Chemicals, preservatives, additives, chemically altered sugars, stripped nutrients, cooking sprays and monosodium glutamate AKA "natural flavors".

3. **Constant Vaccination** - Source: Pharmaceutical companies.

4. **Industrial Dyes** - Sources: Clothing, sheets, comforters, paints, carpets, and countertops.

5. **Modern Cleaners** - Sources: Toothpaste, deodorant, soap, bathroom cleaners, and kitchen cleaners.

6. **Polluted Air** - Sources: US Government chemical trails, automobile exhaust, factory/manufacturing fumes.

7. **STRESS! [Real Reason]** - Sources: All of the above. This is more specifically physical stress or physiological stress.

All of the above topical reasons for cancer are pretty much self-explanatory. On the other hand, the last one it is the most important if you want to avoid cancer in your lifetime: STRESS! I want you to notice that I keep capitalizing the word STRESS. It's that important.

Ask yourselves...why are people dying at 38 years old!? My own brother had a stroke at the age of 36 years old and thank goodness, he's still alive. At the time, I broke down. I nearly quit my job because I wanted to go back and be by his side. My little bro' was dying and there was nothing I could do. Good thing, he is alive, well and doing just fine today. I think all of my immediate family were about to lose it. It was my Dad and Mom that kept everything under control with the entire family. I sincerely believe all the positive thoughts and prayers are the sole motive for my brother's outstanding recovery.

I want to give this particular topic some real thought. I know in most of our minds, we want to live to 100 years old. If we really think about it, it's just an arbitrary number. I don't particularly want to live to 100 years old just to say I've made it there. I want to live a full, healthy life for as long as I can live it!

If I've done everything that I wanted to do with his life and I've accomplished everything that I had set as a goal, then did I not live a full life? With all due respect, the number is irrelevant. I believe sincerely, that it's the level of happiness that you achieve throughout your life that makes it worth the time you spent here. In case you do want to extend your existence on this spinning, blue ball, here are some interesting numbers for you to fathom.

The average lifespan for the normal American is 78.6 years old now. You might ask, "What's wrong with that?" First of all, a human being should easily be able to live to 120 years old. Geneticists would concur with this last statement. The real problem with the number that is given above is that it's lower than the previous two years, which is unheard of! The years 2015 and 2016 are the only years since 1993 that the average age of an American citizen has gone down.

You see, in 1993 we had a dip in life expectancy due to special circumstances. Those being an abnormally high homicide rate, the wide spread of AIDS throughout the country, and an unusual incidence of people dying from freak accidents. That all came to a head in one strange year. Fast forward to today, we have two years where none of these things happened, yet our life expectancy has dropped 2 years straight!

Are you getting worried yet? If not, maybe the reason that these numbers are changing will change your mind. There have been a record amount of heart disease-related problems, strokes, and respiratory-related diseases that have caused a dramatic uptick in deaths among Americans. I knew that would get you a little stirred up. I don't like to see these numbers any more than you do, but I have a very strong suspicion that it has to do with the 7 things that I've labeled above that cause cancer.

I often study the work of a brilliant man who's given extremely accurate insights into the causes of most human conditions that plague our society today. His name is Dr. Robert Morse! Both he and I agree that the number one cause of cancer is #7 on my list: STRESS! By the way, my list isn't in any particular order.

Now, take stress and combine it with the other six factors that I've included on my list above and I think you'll see there is no other outcome for your body other than disease. I think you all would agree that celebrities have access to the best of everything. They have access to the best doctors, the best foods, the best vacations to relieve stress, and no worries about where money is going to come from. After all, they can visit holistic retreats, shop at Whole Foods to buy unlimited organic foods without flinching, and visit the doctor at any time as many times as they would like without having to worry about the bill. I'd say that this is a distinct advantage.

Even with all of the above being true, we still see an alarming number of celebrities dying at extremely young ages. Since we are talking about cancer and this particular chapter, let me mention a few people you might know who have lost their lives to cancer way too early...

Bob Marley: Lung and brain cancer (death age: 37)

Linda McCartney: Breast cancer (death age: 56)

George Harrison: Lung cancer (death age: 58)

Steve Jobs: Pancreatic cancer (death age: 56)

Donna Summer: Lung Cancer (death age: 68)

Bernie Mac: Cancer (death age: 50)

Patrick Swayze: Pancreatic cancer (death age: 57)

Christopher Hitchens: (Author): Cancer (death age: 62)

Stuart Scott: Appendix cancer (death age: 49)

Elizabeth Montgomery (Bewitched): Colorectal cancer (death age: 62)

I personally admire the people that appear on this list who are dead now. I have no doubt that they lived full and exciting lives during their lifetimes. The big question I have for you is, do you think any of them wanted to die at the age that they did? The ages that I have for the death of each of these celebrities is rather low for a human being in any respect. Remember the median age for the average American? It was 79 years old. None of the people on this list made it.

You would think that with me being a 40-year-old man, I'd be worried about death coming for me, especially after looking at this list. Consequently, I have no such worries at all! When you know the nature of your enemy, there is no reason to fear...and cancer is not a fear for me! Since you are reading this book, you know what I know which is: cancer cells are your body's own cells. There's no reason to be afraid of them because they are part of you. These cells became cancerous and therefore, can become healthy again.

There are two types of cancers that reside in our bodies. One type of cancer is an overgrowth of normal healthy cells. The other type of cancers I call black-cell cancers (BCCs).

The first cancer I mentioned are completely healthy cells, however, they get in the way of normal healthy body processes. For example, if these were to block a pathway in our brain, we could have an episode where we'd stop breathing.

The BCCs are the ones that we are most afraid of. Black cell cancers often kill live cells next to the dead cells inside our bodies. They actually feed off of them. This will cause the population of our healthy cells to diminish to the point of no return. Once we've passed this point, we are now in a state of disease that will ultimately kill us if we don't do anything about it.

How can stress cause cancer? It's pretty easy to see how the other 6 adjuvants that appear on the list above can cause cancer. They are self-explanatory. However, stress is a bit of an enigma. Here's how it works: whenever we are stressed, our body produces cortisol. Cortisol is known as the stress hormone. Now don't get this backwards, cortisol does not cause stress, it actually relieves it.

Cortisol is the most powerful anti-inflammatory known to man and it works extremely well and extremely quickly. However, because cortisol only comes in small spurts and in short supply, it will require your body to "steal" precursors from other body parts to produce more cortisol. This will definitely result in hypothyroidism, Cushing's syndrome, panhypopituitarism, and/or enlarged thyroid gland. All of which impact your ability to fight cancer, and regulate your metabolism for delivery of hormones.

In old medical books, they mentioned something called the Stress Triad. In this Triad, your body goes into increasing levels of ineffectiveness as far as function. As indicated by the name, there are three levels. In level 1, we see increased blood pressure, sweaty skin surfaces, and a raised level of anxiety. This is referred to as eustress, or healthy stress. This allows our brains to thrive to accomplish a goal.

However, any level after this one will result in degradation of our physiology. During level 2, these symptoms increase in intensity and along with them come consistent high blood pressure, consistent high cholesterol, migraine headaches, decreased digestive function, and decreased hormone production.

Progressing to the last stage includes bodily breakdown exhibiting heart deformation (from lack of nutrients and hormones), ulcers (holes) in our digestive tract, and decreased liver function. A decrease in liver function is both dangerous and life-threatening. Our livers perform over 500 functions inside the body, all of which are vital to our survival.

Let's go just a bit further here, now add in the other six components of how we get cancer. We are already bombarded with stress which is literally tearing down our body. Add on top of that industrial lubricants, chemical-laden food, vaccines, electromagnetic fields, deadly cleaning supplies, and chemicals being sprayed throughout the air on a daily basis! There is no other conclusion to come to: CANCER!

Whew! I hope that explanation wasn't too long for you. How about I tell you some ways that you can get rid of this cancer instead of going on and on about how it can kill you.

Sound good? Okay!

Section Two

Killing Cancer Naturally

Secret #4: Fire Away, Scotty!

I hope you all got that line from one of my favorite old television shows, 'Star Trek'. It was always a joy watching James T. Kirk fire off his cheesy lines on that basic, almost unbearably cheap studio set. He got the alien girls, he commanded the Starship Enterprise, and his hair was epic. If it weren't for William Shatner's overacting in the series, I doubt if there'd be a 'Star Trek' on television for us to enjoy in syndication. Bottom line...he was a hero! That is what I want to talk to you all about in this chapter: HEROES.

You may not have heard of the man that I'm about to tell you of, however, if you live in Texas, I think you've heard quite a bit about this brilliant doctor. He's been fighting to cure cancer-ridden patients since 1977. His name is Stanislaw Burzynski. Even though his research runs more along the traditional lines of medicine, he has come up with new and innovative ways of treating stage-4 cancers, that are otherwise a death sentence.

Any doctor worth his white jacket should always consider all the alternatives when treating you for any kind of metabolic disease. Since we practice allopathic medicine here in the Western World of the United States, that notion seems to be dying off pretty quickly. I will say this again, there is nothing wrong with going to a hospital, clinic, or medical office if you have an emergency. However, if you are visiting the doctor on a regular basis, you are in for a shortened life!

Dr. Burzynski is one of the better physicians to ever step on Texas soil. He does not advocate patients get any surgeries or treatment before they have gone home and tried to change their diet, their lifestyle, and less invasive procedures to get rid of their cancer. After he has exhausted all of those avenues, then he goes to his special procedure, better known as antineoplastons. Coincidentally, that is the reason that I've named this chapter 'Fire Away, Scotty!' Antineoplastons are injected into the body as a gene-based therapy to directly kill cancer cells using your own bodies genetics to do so. Isn't that cool!?

At present, Dr. Burzynski is getting 25 - 35% cure rates with patients who have late-stage, terminal cancers! You might be asking yourself, is that good? Hell yes it's good! As far as patient getting better (reversing their cancer, but not completely cured), he is closer to a 95% success rate. If you don't know by now, the success rate of chemotherapy and radiation to cure any kind of cancer, not to mention stage 4 cancer, is 3%. You know what else has a 3% success rate with cancer patients? A sugar pill! At this point, you should be asking yourself...why? Why would the government and pharmaceutical companies gang up on Dr. Burzynski to try and criminalize him so they could steal his patents, then shut down his research so that chemotherapy, surgery, and radiation are the prevalent "norm" for these types of procedures? I think you know the answer to this, but we'll talk about that in a later chapter.

If you've heard nothing about this story, Stanislaw is currently fighting the Texas Medical Board in order to be able to save people's lives. I can't believe you have to ask for permission to do this nowadays, as Americans have become so weak about protecting their own liberties!

Even though Dr. Burzynski has saved many late-stage cancer patients with his antineoplaston treatment, he brings up an excellent point. You can't save everyone! Even with the best of cancer cures, there will always be the individualized genetics, chemistry, and tissue make up from different human beings. Yes, no one treatment can cure everyone. Sometimes it seems that Americans are waiting for the magic pill to come down the pipeline to save everyone's life who has cancer. I'm here to tell you, that will never happen!

If you all would like to get caught up on how the United States government tried to railroad Dr. Burzynski, there is a riveting documentary on Netflix you can watch to get yourself up to speed. I've never seen the government partner with pharmaceutical companies to try to stand in the way of progress, and that progress is saving people's lives. Scumbaggery!

Section Two

Killing Cancer Naturally

Secret #5: It's a Rough Ride Down

I'm just wondering, how many of you have Bragg apple cider vinegar in your kitchen at home? Every time I asked this question to my class, most of my students raised their hands and say...YES! I had to wonder to myself, how did all my students find out about the wonderful benefits of apple cider vinegar. After all, there is no public-broadcast news story telling all of us that apple cider vinegar is the best thing since leafy green vegetables. So how did all my students, and probably some of you, find out about the miraculous healing powers of apple cider vinegar?

Diabetes. Recent Studies have shown a definitive link between apple cider vinegar and low blood sugar levels. In one study, participants took 2 tablespoons of apple cider vinegar before bed and saw their blood sugar dropped 4 to 6% by the time they woke up. The blood-lowering effect of the acid in the apple cider vinegar is what helps with insulin sensitivity.

Weight Loss. Drinking apple cider vinegar can make you feel more satiated (full). It has been found that acetic acid inside a CV actually slows fat accumulation. If it's too difficult for you to take apple cider vinegar straight, then added to water or juices if you prefer to drink it. If you prefer to mix it with something, I recommend putting it in the salad dressing food with.

Lower Cholesterol. I think some of you know my position on lowered cholesterol. This is arbitrary science put out there with no scientific backing as to why lower cholesterol helps us. However, there are studies backing up ACV. The journal for Agricultural and food chemistry did a study that showed some very interesting things about apple cider vinegar. Lower back fat even while consuming a high cholesterol diet for the results. Of course, ACV detoxifies our bodies.

Digestive Aid. Do you have severe stomach or abdominal pain? You can start sipping on some diluted apple cider vinegar to help relieve your digestive issues. Because it is a natural antibiotic (killing bacteria), It is able to kill unwanted bacteria in the digestive tract. Some reports that the pectin and apple cider vinegar also helps with intestinal spasms.

Sore Throat. With the above information about digestion and apple cider vinegar fighting bacteria, you should have guessed it can kill bacteria anywhere in the body. That includes your throat. Just mix half apple cider vinegar with half water and gargle for five minutes. Repeat this procedure as needed.

Sinus Issues. Apple cider vinegar as an emulsifier, which means it breaks up mucus in the body. Due to the antibacterial strength of apple cider vinegar, you can use it as part of a nasal wash to get rid of sinus infections. If the nasal wash is a bit too much for you, then warm apple cider vinegar mixed with water. One 8-ounce glass of water plus one tablespoon of apple cider vinegar.

More Energy Please. This is one of my favorite uses for ACV and it might be for you athletes as well. If you're drinking Monster, Rockstar, Red Bull, or any of the chemical-filled energy boosters to get more "pep" out of your day, I want you to throw all of them in the trash right now! The potassium and enzymes inside a CD will do way more for your energy level than any energy drink. One 8-ounce glass of water plus 1 tablespoon of ACV. There are also amino acids contained in this miracle tonic that help combat lactic acid build-up during and after your workout. If you want to have more powerful, effective workout sessions, then this will be your best friend.

Sunburned Skin/Itchy Skin. Apple cider vinegar is also very quick and effective in relieving itchy skin. All you have to do is directly apply apple cider vinegar to the site of itchiness, and feel the irritation go away! This is excellent for bug bite, poison ivy, jellyfish stings, or bee stings. As far as sunburns go, soak in a bath with 1 cup of apple cider vinegar to help ease the discomfort.

Wart Remover. Store-bought wart creams are never a good option when trying to get rid of warts. They are laced with chemicals and preservatives. Another harmful alternative would be going to the doctor. If you're into sadomasochism, then I'd suggest you go into your local doctor's office and let him cut off your warts with an expensive laser or worse yet, slice you up with a scalpel to remove those warts, which will ultimately come back because the root cause was never addressed. Instead, follow this protocol: Soak cotton balls in apple cider vinegar. Then, cover all the warts completely with the cotton balls. Hold the cotton balls in place with tape, then leave them overnight. Do this every night until the warts fall right off! To further speed this process, you can also drink apple cider vinegar at the same time you are performing this protocol.

Detox. ACV Can quickly promote circulation and detoxify our livers. Apple cider vinegar can also bind to toxins to carry deadly impurities out of our body. This will also help clear out the lymphatic system, being that ACV is an emulsifier. One of the biggest benefits of using this is apple cider vinegar acts as a whole-body alkalizer. Bringing your blood to a slightly basic level makes it almost impossible for cancer to exist in your body!

Other Uses. If you want to get rid of most of the chemicals that ARE exposing you and your children to a toxic overload, then use ACV for these daily routines…

Deodorant: Full strength - Wipe on the underarms. The smell goes away after it dries.
Fading Bruises: Full strength - Dap on the bruise, as needed.
Whiten Teeth: 2 parts water/1part ACV - Swish around in the mouth for 5 minutes. Then brush normally.
Mouthwash: 2 parts water/1part ACV - Swish around in the mouth for 5 minutes.

<u>Foot Odor</u>: Full strength - Soak a paper towel in ACV, then wipe your feet thoroughly with the towel. This will balance the pH of your feet to eliminate the odor. The smell goes away after it dries.

<u>Kills Weeds</u>: Full strength - Put in a spray bottle and go nuts!

<u>House Cleaner</u>: 1 part ACV/1 part water - Clean anything and don't worry, the smell goes away after it dries.

<u>Hair Rinse</u>: ⅓ cup ACV to 4 cups of water. Rinse with this AFTER shampooing. Then rinse with cold water. This will remove chemical product from your hair, leaving a nice body and shine. In addition, this will balance your scalp's pH level.

<u>Facial Cleanser</u>: 1 part ACV/1 part water - In combination with balancing your skin's pH, this will also prevent breakouts. If this mixture is too harsh for your skin, use more water.

Cancer Protocol. It's really this simple…

- ✓ **One 8 oz. glass of purified/filtered water**
- ✓ **One tablespoon of apple cider vinegar**
  *Mix and drink.
  *Take every day: once upon waking and once before bed.

OK! I've packed just about all I can get into this chapter. I might have gone a little overboard with giving you useful information, but I don't believe you can ever get too much of a good thing. I'll see you in the next chapter where we'll be talking about some more space-age stuff that you can use to battle any kind of cancer.

See you there.

Section Two

Killing Cancer Naturally

Secret #6: Radio Flyers

No, no, no. This chapter is not about some movie about a flying wagon made in 1992! I know some of you thought it was the height of cinematic brilliance to see a kid's wagon take off and fly into the air with wings too small to even lift a squirrel off the ground, but hey, it was the 90's. *LOL*

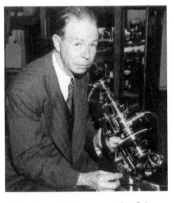 In this chapter, I'm not going to talk to you about a Radio Flyer, per se. I'm going to talk to you about radio waves flying through the air. I hope that's a close enough analogy for some of you English buffs out there. You see, in the 1930's, a microbiologist by the name of **Dr. Royal Rife** (seen on your left) came up with a quite clever solution to getting rid of cancer. His methods did not involve lotions, potions, or anything the like. His methods involved beam frequencies. If that isn't one of the coolest things you've ever heard of, I think you're reading the wrong book. Just kidding, keep reading.

Get this… Dr. Rife came up with the idea to cure cancer with the use of HIGH frequency beams and enlisted the help of an engineer in the summer of 1936 named Philip Hoyland. Hoyland built the high frequency beam machines for Dr. Rife backed by Dr. Rife's science. This marvel of modern science was called a Beam Ray Clinical Instrument. Some proponents of the time didn't think that this name for his epic medical machine had enough cachet. Thus, his high-frequency machines were dubbed Rife Rays! Through the many iterations of his technology, Dr. Rife improved upon his technology. Therefore, each iteration had its own number. It wasn't until version #5 that he found ultimate success in curing cancer on the highest of levels.

Now here's the interesting part, there are different frequencies that Dr. Rife set for different diseases in order to target that particular condition with his methods. Take a look at some of the frequencies below that I found you might find quite interesting.

| Microorganisms | John Crane's 1950's MORs | Rife's M.O.R Frequencies | | | | |
| | | Rife's MORs 1936-1950 | Rife's MORs 1935-1936 | Rife's MORs from 1935 and before | | |
	Frequency in Hz Square Wave	Frequency in Hz Sine Wave	Rife Ray # 4 in Hz Sine Wave	#1 Frequency in Hz Sine Wave	#2 Frequency in Meters Sine Wave	Meters to Hz Sine Wave
1. Actinomycosis (Streptothrix)	784	7,870	192,000	678,000	1,607	186,554
2. Anthrax			139,200	900,000	1,100	272,539
3. Anthrax Symptomatic				400,000	18,000	16,655
4. B. Coli (Rod form)	800	8,020	417,000	683,000	943	317,914
5. B. Coli (Filterable virus)	1552	17,220	770,000	8,581,000	27	11,103,424
6. Bacillus X Filter passing (Cancer - carcinoma)	2128	21,275	1,604,000	11,780,000	17.6	17,033,662
7. Bacillus Y (Cancer - sarcoma)	2008	20,080	1,604,000	11,780,000	17.6	17,033,662
8. Bubonic Plague				160,000	585	512,466
9. Catarrh				1,600,000	175	1,713,100
10. Cholera Spirillum				851,000	312	960,873
11. Contagious Conjunctivitis				1,206,000	148	2,025,625
12. Diptheria				800,000	275	1,090,154
13. Glanders				986,000	407	736,591
14. Gonorrhea	712		233,000	600,000	1,990	150,649
15. Influenza				1,674,000	154	1,946,704
16. Leprosy	600	6,000		743,000	1,190	251,926
17. Pneumonia	776	7,660		1,200,000	785	381,901
18. Spinal Meningitis			427,000	927,800	167	1,795,164
19. Staphylococcus Pyogenes Aureus	728	7,270	478,000	998,740	540	555,171
20. Staphylococcus Pyogenes Albus					546	549,070
21. Streptococcus Pyogenes	880	8,450	720,000	1,214,000	142	2,111,214
22. Syphilis (Treponema Pallidum)	660	6,600	789,000	900,000	108	2,775,856
23. Tetanus	120	1,200	234,000	700,000	19,000	15,779
24. Tuberculosis (Rod form)	803	8,300	369,000	583,000	554	541,142
25. Tuberculosis (Virus form)	1552	16000				
26. Typhoid Fever (Rod form)	712	6,900	760,000	900,000	345	868,964
27. Typhoid Fever (Filter passing)	1862	18,620	1,445,000	9,680,000	21.5	13,943,835
28. Worms		2400				

(RoyalRife.com)

The chart above is just to show you some of the diseases that can be cured using this method and the frequencies required to cure them. This is Earth-breaking stuff from 'Star Trek' that we only thought could happen in a TV show! However, back in 1938, Royal Rife actually sent high frequency beams through human beings' bodies to heal all types of conditions.

Now this is what takes Dr. Rife's intelligence and ingenuity to another level! Initially, he had problems curing the diseases to the extent of success he wanted due to frequency. He thought the problem was the frequencies. Nonetheless in short order, his microbiology background kicked in and his observation of the cell gave him the answer he was looking for.

All of us who went through eighth-grade science class know a human cell has a membrane. The membrane carries a different frequency than the rest of the cell. In looking at this almost rudimentary observation, he came up with the solution he was looking for. There had to be two frequencies administered to the cell in order to fix it correctly. Once the second high beam frequency was added to his therapies, cancers dissolved in no time. Some patients' cancers went away as quickly as weeks!

One frequency is needed to "open" the cell membrane, while the other is able to affect the cancerous portions of our cells without interrupting the functions of the cell. This was a scientific breakthrough which should have been yelled from the mountain tops! Instead, the overwhelming success and notoriety of Dr. Rife's accomplishments caused his work to be driven underground, as his methods were discredited by the "puppet show", AKA the media!

I know some of you might be anxious to pick up one of these machines. Well, a word of caution. Today's so-called "Rife Rays" are anything but. You'll notice in the beginning of this chapter, I highlighted the word "HIGH" in regards to the frequency required to get rid of bodily cancers. This is paramount in getting the results you desire. Most machines claiming to be "Rife Rays" (Rife Beam Rays) are LOW frequency, lacking the power to rid us most disease destroyed by this technology in the 1930's. You'll have to look a little harder to find the HIGH frequency beam rays, but they are out there. Just don't ask me where to look. I'm more along the line of diet, supplementation, and mind power cures all!

I have to say though, I'm up to try anything once. I lied...I might try a few times! *LOL*

On to the next chapter.

Section Two

Killing Cancer Naturally

Secret #7: "The Best Part of Waking Up…"

I'm sure all you coffee drinkers out there where quite excited to see the title for *this* chapter! Of course, the above phrase for "Secret #7" is part of one of the most effective advertising campaigns in commercial history: Folgers Coffee. If you don't remember, the slogan goes, "The best part of waking up (pause) is Folgers in your cup." Wow, you all remember that?! I can't blame you, sometimes, I want to forget it and it still gets stuck in my head. Those circular, electrical, neural signal pathways are something else!

Naturally, I can't leave out the rest of you who are hardcore when it comes to coffee. Some of you like it black and hard! Stop thinking dirty, this is not a Cara McKenna novel. *LOL* Some of you may be able to summon from your memory the ghost of Juan Valdez. You "young'uns" out there may not know this reference, but Juan Valdez is NOT a real person.

This is a coffeehouse chain which brings us the freshest coffee beans from the high-reaching hills of

Columbia! I've found this is actually true! This chain did originate in Columbia and grows one of the best grades of coffee in the world created by Colombia's National Association of Coffee Growers. Talk about interesting, especially to you coffee heads. I'm hoping this next statement doesn't sound strange, but I don't think I can avoid the weirdness of this next bit of information.

This section does have everything to do with coffee, but NOT drinking it. It's about shooting it into your butt! Yes! Coffee in your anus. Wait! I don't want anyone blowing scolding, hot coffee into their backside. This should not turn into a trip to the emergency room. Right now, I'll take you into why this is important, then give you the exact regiment. You'll be able to clean up your body's life force in no time. In fact, you may be singing my new slogan, "The best part of waking up (pause) is Folgers in your BUTT!" I love it.

Some of you may not know this, but your liver performs over 500 functions! Because of this, we have to take extremely good care of our most regenerative organ. I want you to really think about this: if your brain were completely dead, the rest of your body could still live and perform some of its most vital functions. However, if our liver where to stop functioning, we die! Plain and simple.

For a lot of you, I don't think you get the gravity of what your liver does for you. Allow me to expound. You take in toxins from every conceivable entry point of your body. Via our lungs, we inhale pollutants and carcinogens directly from the air. Through our skin, we take in poisons from soaps, deodorant, toothpaste, and for you ladies, one of the deadliest compounds known to absorb into the skin and cause bodily problems: make-up! Even our colon takes a huge beating from the poisons that we ingest like carrageenan, soy lecithin, MSG, and trans-fats.

Ironically, our body tries to put the poisons out of our systems via the same exact pathways! You see, from your kidneys you get rid of waste via urine, our colons help us get rid of waste via feces, and our lungs help us expel carbon dioxide as well as gaseous poisons from our bodies.

I know what some of you are thinking, you're thinking, "If my liver already has everything taken care of, then I have nothing to worry about. Right?" Wrong! Our liver is actually collecting toxins and other additives, preservatives, chemicals, and poisons we ingest on a daily basis. Sometimes as far back as when we were 1 year old! I don't know any better reason to clean our liver other than doing what I suggest above, which is a coffee enema.

Previously, I referred to a "life force". With those two words, I was referring to our liver, which performs over 500 functions within our bodies. If you want to know just some of the crucial missions our liver carries out, here are a few: immunity against infection, a factory for proteins and cholesterol, excretes waste through bile, regulates blood clotting, clears our blood of drugs, chemicals, and alcohol, converts excess glucose to starch for storage, and breaks down fat for digestion. Keep in mind, that's only 7 of the functions that your liver performs. So, you can imagine how significant this bodily organ is to us.

Do any of your friends drink alcohol? I don't think I know any of my friends who don't. You may recall, your blood does not clot very well when you are drunk. Why? It may be because your alcohol-cleansing liver is trying to keep you alive, after all, we did mention it regulates blood clotting in our bodies as well. It's almost as if the benefits never stop.

Now that you weekend "wine warriors" have a good handle on what the liver does, there is no excuse for continuing to kill it with fermented alcoholic beverages. However, I am not the government, so live your life anyway that you want to. After all, I am not the FDA and am not going to come to your house with guns drawn to make sure you don't do it!

Let's get down to some more serious matters of history, and explain to you why coffee enemas are extremely important. I already let you know that they actually flush your liver of toxins, but why coffee? Some gurus online will actually say to use something else. They say to use water only, they say to use baking soda and water, and they also advocate you using Himalayan sea salt in some instances. I'm ashamed to admit it, but I've tried all of these. They all feel the same. I have suffered no adverse side effects and no disruption of my system or its normal function.

There's only one problem I have with the above solutions, and that's that they are not stimulants. The above-mentioned alternatives do alkalize the tissues around your rectal area. So, I have no problem with them. On the other hand, coffee does so much more! Coffee's one glaring benefit over the rest of these methods is that coffee is a stimulant. The former alternative methods will only enter the liver then flush *some* of the toxins from the liver, leaving some behind. Alternatively, organic ground coffee in combination with purified filtered water will enter the liver, expand the liver, stimulate the tissues, and drain *all* the toxins from your liver from decades of buildup!

A Home-Based Therapy

Why do I stand firmly behind this? Well, even if you don't believe that coffee is the best method for getting toxins out of your liver, you can't disagree with one thing...the Gerson Therapy! In 1881, a special human being was born into this world that was meant to save lives. His name was Max Gerson. This German-born scientist and later physician, started curing tuberculosis cases as early as the 1920s, consistently. In 450 of the worst cases of tuberculosis that turned out to be terminal, Dr. Gerson actually completely cured 446 of the 450 patients! By this success standard alone, I would have to say that coffee enemas, which were a main part of his therapy, are nothing short of a miracle.

Dr. Max Gerson believed in a diet based approach to healing as a therapy. I must say, I wholeheartedly agree with Dr. Gerson and all of his medical research he's put forward throughout the decades. One thing that stood out to me about Dr. Gerson was his ability to heal terminal illnesses, some of which he found he could heal by accident. His specialty was tuberculosis, however, he found that other serious, even deadly, diseases would go away using his diet-based therapy. Some of these included body-wide tumors and late-stage cancer metastases.

I will spare you the long, boring details of the information found in his clinical trials. I do want you to know, however, if you would like to see details on how well these treatments worked in real life case studies, I would suggest you pick up a book called 'A Cancer Therapy: Results Of 50 Cases'. In this book, Dr. Gerson outlines some of his most difficult cases and how they turned out. I often refer to the book, and use some of this detailed remedies for people I help.

Leaning on my experience, there is no better method than to treat serious and terminal diseases with a diet based program. Most people in our country today believe taking medications on a daily basis is what maintains health. They are sorely mistaken! ABSENCE OF SYMPTOMS DOES NOT EQUAL GOOD HEALTH!

You see, my training as a root cause analysis specialist won't allow me to believe in allopathic medicine. Allopathic medicine is the treatment of symptoms by use of surgery, radiation, and chemicals but never taking care of what actually caused the disease or condition.

[Let's take an example]

You go into the doctor for back pain...this isn't a prescription-triggering event, but the doctor prescribes for you 500 mg of ibuprofen per day. You say, "Sounds good, Doc. Thanks!" After a good 6 to 8 weeks of feeling "OK", you go back because the pain has returned (IE Your body built a tolerance to the medication). Speedier than the fastest gun in the West, he whips out his handy pad and shoots you another prescription. Hold on, but this time, it's for

1000mg. He has to up the dose in order for your body to respond. Now, you're happy again!

However, over the next two weeks, you notice your ankles are sore, your neck is stiffening, and your hip joints ache. What's going on? You trek back to the physician's office and exclaim, "Doc, I'm having body-wide aches and pains. Do you know what's happening?" The doctors say, "These are just signs of aging, and nothing to worry about, but it does involve pain. Tell you what, I'll give you something to ease this transition. Go have this filled out immediately!" You have a brand-new prescription for one of the most powerful muscle-pain killers on the market, Codeine.

You are being a very good patient to this point, taking all the doctor's recommendations. You sincerely believe, you'll get better. The next day, you pick up your new prescription to "ease" your muscle pain. Little did you know that you'd be right back in his medical office for abdominal pain 3 months later. These pains are so severe and sharp in intensity, you can't sleep since they started.

Since this is causing a noticeable change in your lifestyle, the doctor (being the good guy he is) will take you off the Codeine, and put you on Demerol, another super-strong pain reliever. Even though, you are not experiencing the migraine headaches that started after the Codeine, you still aren't sleeping that well anymore. So, you go back to your "doc" for another diagnosis on the non-sleep you're getting. He says, "Everything appears to be fine with you, but I'm going to put you on maximum-strength melatonin to help you get some shut-eye. That should do it."

You've added another medication to your arsenal...CONGRATULATIONS! After 2 months, something strange happens. Even though you are taking sleeping pills, you can't sleep! What the f*** happened?! It must be that damned liver again, and you would be right! Your body has built a tolerance once again, thus, calling for the good ole' family doctor to "up" our dosage AGAIN! After a year of tedious doctor visits, chronic misinformation, no feedback, and a staggering bill for medical services, all you have is a medicine store in your bathroom! There isn't even any room for your Johnson and Johnson Q-tips!

[End of example]

I hope you found lots of sarcasm in the above scenario. It's meant to be there and I laid it on pretty thick. On a more serious note, I want you to look at this more closely. For every bottle of medication you have in your medicine cabinet right now, you can expect to cut 5 years off the end of your life! That is not an exaggeration, that is literal.

You might have heard of a man named Bruce Lee. He is the Kung Fu Master! Most people thought Bruce Lee would die in the fight of his life (which he trained every day for). However, it was not a spectacular, death-defying street fight that took his life. Unfortunately, it was drugs!

He took a regiment of herbs called Kashish. They were extremely powerful, health-promoting herbs but they do cause severe stomach cramps. One night before a movie shoot, Bruce needed to take a nap because of an excruciating headache. He borrowed a sleeping pill from one of his fellow colleagues. A contraindication occurred, poisoning this elite-level fighter. He never woke from that nap!

You might have heard of this kinda good dancer named Michael Jackson. The King of Pop didn't die at a ripe old age and have his grandchildren around his bed. MJ died in his sleep from over medication prescribed by a doctor who was forced to give it to him.

You may have also heard of a woman named Whitney Houston. This pop singer was once dubbed the most talented singer of any generation! In her prime, I would have to agree. Whitney Houston also did not die at a tender, elderly age like you would think most successful celebrities would. She died by drowning in a hotel bathtub due to paralysis from having too many medications in her system mixed with alcohol!

To a lot of the American public, taking over-the-counter, prescription, and illicit drugs seems like just another thing that celebrities do in order to deal with their overwhelmingly hectic lives. We're even dismissive of these terrible acts.

To me, I see rich people who have been trained to go to others to solve their problems. When they are told to do something, they do it. I'm sure if you look back on your life, you will see that you have done exactly the same thing, as I have. We trust doctors with our health believing that they are the holders of all knowledge and have our best interests at the forefront of their minds. I have found through disappointing experience, that is not the case!

While you let the doctor medicate you for one symptom after the other, their office only gets more profitable. I thought the purpose of a doctor's office was to make you well. Now I see that's just a quaint notion meant for the past.

You are now a lead in advertising system that counts you as a number. It reminds me of an episode of 'The Twilight Zone' called the 'Obsolete Man'. That was in 1961, yet, it holds true for 2017! This enrages me to no end. People are not f****ing leads, numbers, or stats. They are human beings DAMN IT!

The Coffee Enema Protocol

Here is the part you've been waiting for (or dreading) in order to cleanse your liver, flush those toxins, and cleaning your blood as if you had a brand, spanking new liver. For all practical purposes, you will! Just follow this procedure…

How To Perform The Coffee Enema (Video on my channel):

Step #1: Get yourself some organic "enema" whole coffee beans. You can get these from any health food store or from Amazon.

Step #2: Grind the coffee in a coffee grinder to produce a fine coffee powder for adequate absorption.

Step #3: Boil 1 Liter of purified water for 5 to 7 minutes. Do not use tap water, it defeats the purpose of this. If you can't obtain purified water, boil tap water for 30 minutes (no less) to rid it of chlorine.

Note: You can buy a ZeroWater ZP-010 10-Cup Pitcher to make tap water purified water, which is free of chlorine and fluoride. This is the Zero water claim.

Step #4: Reduce heat from high to medium-low, then add coffee to the boiling water. Boil coffee water for 10 minutes.

Step #5: Let the coffee mixture cool to just warmer than room temperature. If it's still hot to touch after this time, you may add ice cubes. Pour this mixture into a 1-liter enema bucket. (Kendall Seamless Enema Set with Bucket) or (Stainless Steel Enema Kit 2 Quart Container. No Latex). Make sure the tubing is attached, and the tubing is closed off. Check temperature.

Step #6: Lubricate the tubing end with vegan soap, then insert the tubing anally up to 3 inches. Lie on your **right** side on the bathroom floor. Release the valve on the tubing and allow half the mixture to enter the anus (½ liter). Try to hold for 12 minutes, then release into the toilet. This works better if you have already defecated. Wait a few moments, then drain the rest of the coffee solution into your anus. Try to hold again for 12 minutes. Then void into the toilet. If you can't hold it, don't worry. You'll be able to hold it longer the more often you do this.

*You'll notice that your energy and mood can spike (to say the least) immediately after this. After your coffee enema, you should feel an extreme spike of energy and vitality. You'll also notice that you can now absorb nutrients from your food a lot more quickly. We may also notice that junk food passes through your system in a hurry. You may even surprise your partner in the bedroom. If that ain't enough reason, I don't know what is!

Frequency of Enemas

>The coffee enema should only be done every 5 days to a week. This allows the colon to normalize. (*Exception: If the body is severely toxic (you are really sick), you may do coffee enemas once every two hours for 5 days in a row.*)

>Then one enema every 7 days for 2 months.

>Then one enema every 2 weeks for 3 months.

>Then one enema every month for a year.

>Now you can do one coffee enema per year for life to keep the liver healthy and keep cancer instances to non-existent levels. That is if you don't continue to poison yourself.

Now if you combined this coffee enema procedure with a plant-based diet regime, you'll be able to knockout 98% of diseases, cancers, and conditions that happened to the average North American citizen. That is provided you can stay consistent.

This chapter has only been as long as it has because I believe it is one of the most effective natural remedies that exists today. The mind-blowing part about this therapy is it's been in use and working since the 1920s!

I know you're ready, so let's move on to the next chapter.

Section Two

Killing Cancer Naturally

Secret #8: Taking The White Stuff

Reading the title to this chapter, I know some of you had flashbacks of Tony Montana in Scarface! Doing lines of blow won't get rid of your cancer, but it will make you forget that you ever had it! For those of you who take things literally, please don't go out and start doing lines of cocaine with your BFFs! I don't want an overdose to be the cure of your cancer.

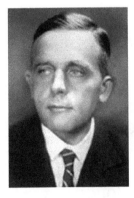

The white stuff I'm talking about is called baking soda (sodium hydrogen carbonate). Yeah, that white stuff that sits in your refrigerator and absorbing odors from all the rancid takeout you left over from last weekend. That's it! Now, I know you're asking yourself "What does baking soda have to do with curing cancer?"

In truth, everything! The distinguished gentleman you are looking at in the photo on your right is Otto Warburg. This 1931 Nobel Prize winner concluded that "...no cancer could exist in an alkaline environment". You may have noticed that there is a huge movement of people drinking alkaline water now-a-days. Some of the products include Real Water, Alkaline Water, and Core Water. All of this H_2O is designed to take your acidity scale to a more basic level.

The whole premise behind this is if you can alkalize your body, then you can prevent any cancer from taking hold in your healthy cells. The good news is this can be done as a preventative measure instead of a last-ditch effort after you've been diagnosed with a late-stage cancer or late-stage diabetes.

The liquid portion of your blood, called plasma, is made up of 91% water. The pH of water is neutral or 7 pH. Anything dropping lower than 7, is considered acidic. Having our blood at acidic levels is one of the worst things we can ask for health wise. Being acidic allows cancers to proliferate throughout our systems using our blood/lymph as a communication device and to spread itself.

However, if our bodies are geared more to the alkaline side, there's almost no chance of cancer destroying our bodily tissues and deteriorating our health. This sounds like a very easy thing to do, until you consider that all of the things you consider as tasting good are on the acidic side. How many of you get up in the morning and start your day with a nice, big, fat, cup of coffee? I'm going to guess a lot of you. Coffee is 4 pH. You just started off your day with a shot of acidity!

There are some anomalies I probably should tell you about. **Tomatoes and lemons** are extremely acidic as they exist outside of the body. However, when lemons and tomatoes touch your stomach acid, they become extremely alkaline, actually becoming very good for you to rid yourself of disease and cancer. So, there is no need to start pulling your hair out because you thought you had to stop eating salsa and guacamole! I feel like a good person now that I've told you that. *LOL*

How about you **women and alkalinity**? Did you know that a woman's entire reproductive system is based on how balanced she can keep her pH? Let me give you a stark example. Women all over the world deal with a pre-menstrual syndrome or PMS. Some women can suffer from a condition called menometrorrhagia. This signifies an abnormally large amount of blood discharge during a woman's monthly cycle. Some woman called it a "heavy flow". Well, this is all determined by an average woman's pH level.

I'm going to give you ladies another reason to use baking soda besides getting rid of cancer, as if that wasn't already good enough. The survival of a woman's fetus inside the uterus during pregnancy is all-important. The environment of the uterus must be suitable in pH level in order for a fetus to survive and flourish. If the pH level drops below 6 or is too acidic, your body's sensors will pick up on this acidity and literally tear out the entire wall to make room for new cells that would be more suitable in pH level. This accounts for the excessive flow during menstruation.

If pregnant, the embryo or fetus would not be able to survive an extremely acidic environment. In rare cases, this will lead to stillbirths and spontaneous abortions. Today, this is becoming all too common.

Drinking soft drinks, drinking alcohol, eating foods laced with additives, preservatives, and chemicals is making this problem accelerate at a deafening paste.

If we look at the other side, when the pH level is neutral or a little alkaline in nature, the emerging fetus thrives quite well during pregnancy. In women who are not pregnant, this tends to create a lighter flow during menstruation. If your uterus reads the internal environment as suitable for having a baby, then there's no need for excessive maintenance. Thus, the menstrual flow is less intense.

REMEMBER, too much of a good thing is a bad thing! Don't over alkalize your system because this has dire effects of its own, one being birth defects. Everything in our bodies is a balance and should be considered as such. We want to strike a balance but slightly to the alkaline side.

The Baking Soda Protocol

Besides the fact that it's extremely effective, it's also one of the easiest protocols to follow in all of medical history! Here are the directions for how to execute alkalizing your system with baking soda. Don't overdo it, just follow the directions…

1 glass of purified/filtered water (8 oz.)
1 tablespoon of 100% pure baking soda (brand is irrelevant)
***Mix the 2 components, then drink.**

*Take this once when you wake and once when you are getting ready for bed. This is ideal for any height-weight combination.

If you need further proof that this very simple concoction can make major changes in your life, I want you to go find real life case studies and ask people who have done this how it worked for them. I don't want you making any assumptions that this will or will not work. I want you to do your own research! I am not writing this book for my health, I'm writing it for yours!

In case you don't know where to start looking for these "case studies", I recommend you go to YouTube so you can see real people doing this on video and showing you exactly how much they use and how it works over time. Search for "cure cancer with baking soda" and see what pops up. You may also want to go even further and find a group of natural cancer survivors who have cured themselves. I use a site called 'Meetup.com' to do this. You can *only* pick up useful information that will aid you in your journey.

Some of you cynics out there may be asking "What's the catch?" I'll tell you in the next chapter.

Section Two

Killing Cancer Naturally

Secret #9: The Catch

You may be thinking, "Yeah, AL! All this junk sounds great, but WHAT'S THE CATCH? What you're telling me is my doctor's full of sh** and I can take care of most of these life-threatening diseases at home on my own?! Come on! I think you're smoking too much of that "Ganja" you were talking about in Chapter 2! Why should I believe you? Who are you to advise me on my health? I like my doctor, and he has been good to my family. I can't just turn my back on him! Well...tell me something. I'm listening!"

Whoa! Some of you all are mean! *LOL* I've got thick skin, so it ain't no thang. First, who am I to give health advice to anyone? Let's see, I'm a 7-year collegiate advanced anatomy and physiology instructor, a practicing medical researcher, and a trained, 6-year root-cause analysis specialist. That's a mouthful. Oh, and if that wasn't "doing it" for you, I don't believe in reading case studies and statistics alone to see if something works. I only rely on REAL-LIFE case studies and methods I've tried on myself and people I've helped that ACTUALLY work! That's all and that's it.

You won't find any theorizing going on with my research! Anything I recommend for you is probably in my cabinet right now or is on its way to my house from Amazon.com. *LOL* I hate to admit that I shop at Amazon a lot but hey, they have the best prices! Amazon almost always has exactly what I'm looking for. I do have to include a caveat here so that you all don't get confused. What works for me and my body will not work for every one of you. Please don't think you will get the same results in the same time and in the same way that I have.

I always have to throw statements, like that last one, into my conversation because there are always some people out there that believe treatments, either holistic or traditional, should work the same way on everyone. That is NOT the case! Every single thing that I mentioned here in this book will work for most people. However, there will always be people who have a different DNA make-up, a strange blood type, or an uncommon chemical makeup.

Occasionally, when you visit your local bookstore, you'll see a book on the shelf that actually tells you how to eat based on your body type. This acknowledges that there are various body styles that you all have and you should construct a diet that is beneficial to your particular body type. Dr. Peter D'Adamo and Catherine Whitney have a book available called 'Eat Right 4 Your Type'. In this book, they conclude that eating for your *blood* type is a much more effective way of losing weight than simply counting calories or any of the other fad diets that are on the market today.

It seems that every day we are learning more and more about our bodies and how food can be used to effectively treat difficult, or even deadly diseases. What I have learned in my studies of the human body have been extraordinarily helpful in turning my life around and helping me to lose almost 50 pounds in the last few years... and keep it off! During this time, I've also gotten my PSA (prostate specific antigen) test all the way down to zero.

I may as well tell you, my dad had an elevated PSA. Needless to say, this was not a great time for my father as it did weigh on his mind as to whether or not he would live or die of prostate cancer. That's a heavy mind trip to put on anybody! Well, me being the offspring of my dad, I went to get mine checked around 32 years old. I thought it may run in the family. Unfortunately, I was right. My PSA level had a reading of 4 nanograms per milliliter, which is considered suspicious. All I can think when the doctor told me this was, "I'm going to die!" One thing I did know after the doctor gave me his diagnosis was simply by telling me about this condition, my immune system would drop almost 30%.

I want you to notice I said "this condition" and not "my condition". The medical industry has done a very good job of getting patients to own their diagnosis. See, if you own the disease, then you'll want to take care of it with the aid of a doctor, of course. When something is yours, you want to take care of it. Right? This is one of the many head games that the traditional Western Medical system plays on its citizens. Taking ownership of your diagnosis will ensure one thing...that you get to keep it!

To continue my story, I was scared to death! All I could think was how short this life is and how I was (now) going to potentially be on medication for the rest of my life. I'm pretty sure this is how my Dad felt. Not one to take direction (or medication), I started looking in medical research books and on the internet for additional information on my condition and how I could get rid of it. I happened to stumble upon a book written by a man mentioned earlier in this book. The text was called 'Healing the Hopeless' and it was written by Dr. Max Gerson! The book spoke to me because at that moment, I really felt hopeless.

After reading this book, all it took was $168 worth of organic groceries, six weeks, and a willingness to stick to a routine involving regular coffee enemas and a daily juicing regiment. Later, I added mineralization to my diet plan to kick my results into overdrive! To this day, I have no PSA reading and I am presently 40 years old. The same can be done for you, provided you have a willingness to better yourself and can stick to a program. Below are some of the things you may read on the internet and that may decrease your overall white blood cell count...

Here are some PSA guidelines from ZeroCancer.Org (https://zerocancer.org/learn/about-prostate-cancer/detection-diagnosis/psa-test/) and how you should monitor them…

In general, a PSA level that is above 4.0 ng/mL is considered suspicious. However, there are many other factors to consider before taking further action. The following are some general PSA level guidelines:

- *0 to 2.5 ng/mL is considered safe*
- *2.6 to 4 ng/mL is safe in most men but talk with your doctor about other risk factors*
- *4.0 to 10.0 ng/mL is suspicious and might suggest the possibility of prostate cancer. It is associated with a 25% chance of having prostate cancer.*
- *10.0 ng/mL and above is dangerous and should be discussed with your doctor immediately. It is associated with a 50% chance of having prostate cancer.*

However, PSA levels can easily rise with greater age. You and your physician should consult age-specific normal PSA ranges.

My advice: Never put any stock into a PSA reading! They are only 23% accurate, at best. If you want to read that backwards, that means they are wrong 77% of the time! In addition to that, 97% of men who have prostate cancer survive! Do you actually believe that you will be one of the 3% who will die of prostate cancer if you don't get it taken care of? I highly doubt it. Stop listening to your doctor and start doing your own research!

When you read information like this on the interwebs, it makes you think there is nothing you can do WITHOUT the help of a physician. My mission in this life is to inform you differently on this matter. Anything that is not an acute emergency, can be fixed, treated, or remedied at home!

The Catch

Have you ever heard the phrase, "What's the catch?" If not, then you might have been taken advantage of a time or two in your life. Just kidding...but not really. *LOL* Anyway, it's meant to suggest that something is "hidden behind the curtain", "the other shoe hasn't dropped", or my favorite cliché, "this is too good to be true!"

Some of you might be thinking, "Ok, Al! What's the catch?" I think I know the questions you're asking in your head, so let's answer them right now...

"You say I can cure cancer without going to the doctor...AND do it from home?!" **Yes!**

"According to you, I can get rid of a stage-4 cancer, which is terminal, and not have to visit a hospital once?!" **Affirmative!**

"I have late-stage diabetes. You believe I can completely reverse this condition, even if it's Type-1 or Type-2 and not have to take insulin for the rest of my life?! **Definitely!**

Wait, wait, wait! The dentist told me I CANNOT grow my adult teeth back. Now you are saying I can?! **Sure can!**

"Ok, one more. Instead of having my thyroid surgically removed at a big hospital, I can treat my thyroid with diet at home and even restore its normal function?! **Yup!**

So, your last question might be, "What's the catch?"

I know the above questions that I've answered in the affirmative are all treatable because I've remedied them on myself and others willing to try my techniques. So, there's absolutely no question, they work! The real question is, can you get your mind to believe that it will actually work for you? Sometimes, we look at someone else's success and believe that it's not possible for us. They must have some kind of supernatural powers or they have some strange, alien DNA they were born with.

From personal experience, none of these cases are special in the least. They are ordinary people, doing everyday things, who actually tried something that I thought might work for them. There are no tricks, gimmicks, or special procedures. Only a willingness to get better. That's all that's required.

The real "catch", if you could call it that, is your very involvement in the system that is killing you in the first place. In my humble opinion, natural and holistic treatments for our bodies does not work as well once we have subjected ourselves to the cut-burn-poison model in modern medicine. Let me give you an example so that this may sit better with you...

According to the modern-day traditional medical system, late-stage cancers and diabetes can only be managed until your death! Treatments are considered only to ease your pain but never to reverse these deadly conditions. The success rates of chemotherapy and radiation are at a dismal 3%! Let me remind you that a sugar pill has the exact same effect on your cancer! Think about that, a placebo has the exact same healing power as a $300 billion medical therapy. Talk about a waste of money!

This is not only the catch, but the catch-22! You believe by going to the doctor, it will extend your life by helping you manage this cancer. Nothing could be further from the truth! Chemotherapy and radiation, along with surgeries to remove tumors, are proven to shorten life, not extend it! The Catch-22 is you are going to a doctor thinking he is attempting to save your life, when in actuality, he's actually shortening it.

The original catch in all of this is when you expose yourself to these purely medieval methods, it severely decreases the effects holistic treatments have on your body!

Case in point, it would normally take an average person who is 5 foot 7 inches and 165 pounds about 12 months to 18 months to rid themselves of a stage-four cancer permanently using only diet and mineralization techniques. On the other hand, if we were to use the traditional Western methods of treating cancer (usually about 10 sessions of chemotherapy and radiation at a cost of about $80,000), then it would take almost 10 years for the holistic treatments to have the same effect!

I know this looks grim but cheer up, all you have to do is keep your ass out of the hospital and you'll be just fine! There is nothing wrong with going to the hospital in case of emergencies, nonetheless, if you are going to the hospital for chronic conditions, there is no need to set foot in a medical prison! Keep this in mind, only sick people visit the hospital. Do you want to be sick all your life?

That's all I have in this section on how to rid your body of cancers and other common medical disease. Take heart, though, there is much more to come in the chapters to follow. I'll see you there.

Section Three

Do You Suffer From Any Of These?

Secret #10: Migraine Headaches

Have you all ever heard of Ben Affleck, Elle MacPherson, Janet Jackson, Carly Simon, Serena Williams, Elvis Presley, Whoopi Goldberg, Cindy McCain, or Lisa Kudrow? You might have. After all, these are extremely well-known celebrities whom dominate screen, runway, and sport. From the outside, it appears that everything is perfect and the world is at their fingertips. To the contrary, there is one other glaring commonality between these famous, public figures...they all suffer from severe migraine headaches!

Before we get too deep into the subject of migraine headaches, you should know that all migraine headaches are not created equal. There are different causes for migraine headaches and there are different types of migraine headaches affecting various parts of the brain. Let's get down to this, there are sinus migraines, hemisphere migraines, cluster migraines, and general dull-pain migraines. As if this buffet of headaches wasn't enough, they all (in some way) disturb the blood vessels, tissue, and coverings of the brain. Needless to say, our nerves become affected by this.

If you keep constant pressure on a nerve, the nerve will die. Migraine headaches provide that consistent pressure. If you thought doing hardcore drugs killed a lot of brain cells, try a migraine on for size. If you are suffering from migraines on a daily or semi-daily basis, you're killing more brain cells than alcohol ever could!

I don't want to get too nerdy on you right now but I do want to let you know a little bit about each one of these types of migraines. The sinus migraine actually stems from an infection of the sinus cavities right behind our eye sockets. On both sides of your head behind your orbits (eye sockets) you have four chambers that we call sinus cavities. Due to nasal infections, these cavities become infected by bacteria most of the time, causing irritation to the nerves running to these cavities, thus, causing irritation in the brain. With these type of headaches, it feels like our eyeballs are being pushed right out of there sockets!

Hemisphere migraines are a different animal altogether. Even though the pain is just as great as with sinus migraines, with hemisphere migraine headaches the pain is only on one side of the head. Here's the freaky part, because hemisphere migraines are only on one side of the head, they can move to the other side of the head, literally feeling like something is burrowing from one side to the other inside your skull! Hemisphere migraines are usually the result of what we call a cerebral depression, a disturbance that spreads over the cerebrum causing brain-wide inflammation.

Let's get into cluster migraine headaches for just a moment. Cluster migraines are caused by the exact same things as the other migraines, however, cluster migraines are usually localized around the eye. This localization can be around both eyes. This type of migraine usually brings on one of the worst kinds of pains that seems like a sharp, then dull pain that results in a dimming of vision. When your vision is blurred, dimmed, or made sensitive to light, you can bet that your occipital lobe is inflamed.

Lastly, we come to general, dull-pain migraine headaches. These headaches are the most common and usually result in a dull pain and a slight sensitivity to light which brings on more of a headache later. This headache, since it is brain-wide, is most likely to lead to nausea and vomiting. Irritation of the neurons of the brain is the blame for this one too.

Just a side note here, anytime your brain is being injured, whether it be from a headache or trauma, nausea and vomiting are the most common symptoms to denote brain injury.

What's The Cause?

Vaccines. At some time or another throughout your lifetime, you (and your kids) will be urged to get your vaccines in order to make the population a safer place. If you believe this, then go on believing it. I have no intention of trying to change your mind if your mind cannot be changed. In my research, though, I found that vaccines have awful adjuvants added that affect the brain adversely. The first one I found is called thimerosal (ethyl mercury). The other is called aluminum oxide. You may think that these have no effect in "trace amounts", but you should know that an infant would have to weigh 550 pounds to accommodate the "trace amounts" in ONE shot of the MMR vaccine (Dr. Gary Null, 'Autism - Made In The U.S.A. Documentary). You can imagine the devastation this will have on your brain and body tissue from the normal schedule of vaccines given to children BEFORE one year of age, which equals 69 doses at present (January 2016)!

To be completely fair, not all vaccines have mercury or aluminum oxide in them. On the other hand, most do! So excuse my "French" but BIG F***KIN' WHOOP! I found through my own tedious research that none of the ingredients found in any vaccine are helpful to a human beings tissue or well-being. So why are they putting it in there? I quote "...because it helps it work better" quoted from Merck press release. When these pharmaceutical research studies say these chemicals and preservatives inside vaccines are making it work better, what they mean is it's so harmful to the cell membrane, our body has no choice but to produce antibodies.

Antibodies, in physiology, are called B-lymphocytes. These are memory cells that remember what antigens attacked you so that the next time the invaders comes back, you can more efficiently kill the deadly antigens. The important thing to remember here is antibodies are not formed more quickly simply because you have been vaccinated. Nor does it mean, if you've been vaccinated, that you will not get the disease. So my question is, why are we being injected with vaccines? Let me answer that for you, absolutely NO REASON!

Headache medications. Some of us harbor unhealthy vices. Some that come to mind are smoking, eating, drinking alcohol, and even hardcore drugs like cocaine and heroin. There is no judgment. Do your thing! The fact that you can take a trip without leaving your house is a miracle unto itself. I don't do it but to each his own.

One of the vices not mentioned above is one of constant overuse of prescribed and over-the-counter medications. Whenever we have a pain that pops up in our everyday lives, we reach right for that bottle. That bottle is not alcohol, but a more deadly variety. The medication bottle. Think about that, you don't trust your body enough to fix its own problems. In fact, it's supremely intelligent and knows exactly what to do. However, you've let television commercials and internet ads dictate how you treat your body. I've never seen so many bottles of Aleve, Motrin, Excedrin, or ibuprofen in my life! Not to "put them on blast", but these are just a few problems my students I see on an everyday basis.

If you are taking any of the brands of headache medication mentioned above, these will only mask the pain. The underlying cause is still there, which is why your headaches will continue! You cannot cover a problem with a topical solution and expect the problem to go away. It will never go away!

Being a root cause analysis specialist, I am trained specifically to look for the cause of a problem. Sometimes there are multiple causes to a problem. In those cases, we have to narrow it down to one specific, overriding cause that we can pinpoint and when we solve that, the other problems go away.

The problem with taking painkillers of any type is the tolerance our bodies build to anything foreign being introduced. Our bodies get used to things. Once your brain calculates the amount of drug you're taking, it will rearrange your set points so that the drug does not have the same effect. Once this happens, you have two choices: you'll need a higher dosage to get the same amount of relief or you will have to switch medications so as to confuse your brain, in order to get an effect.

Either way, neither of these methods is good for us. Increasing the dosage on a headache painkiller will only cause more waste products to be produced inside of our body. Once this happens, your body will have no idea how to process them. The only other option is storage of the poison. This is going to occur in your fat cells, which will take any junk or poison that is introduced to them. Not only will this poison enter your fat cells, but it will pool inside of your cartilage and joints.

If you pay close attention, you may notice your joints start to ache after a while of taking any kind of painkiller, whether it be for a headache or any other body pain. I would also be willing to bet that if you got a colonoscopy after 6 months or more of using these "meds", you would develop a condition called "leaky gut". The doctor is going to call them gastrointestinal ulcers on your paperwork, but "leaky gut" sounds more innocent. So they'll tell you that's what you have, then put you on a different medication. I sincerely doubt you want your life to be a series of doctor's visits, pharmacy trips, and life-long surgeries.

Foods. If you've looked at any of my YouTube videos, you know I advocate a plant-based diet along with regular supplementation. Eating a plant-based diet is code for an alkaline diet. Eating foods that reside on the acidic side of the pH scale, unfortunately, create an environment ripe for attack by cancers and disease!

To create a separation in your mind between acidic and alkaline foods, let me give you this small mnemonic to help you remember. Anything that is plant-based is alkaline in nature. Our blood pH is 7. This is considered neutral and the best place to be, as your body's set points are geared towards this pH. If we are a little bit towards the alkaline side, it's almost impossible for disease or cancer to exist in your body.

Looking at the other side though, anything below seven is considered acidic. When acidity is high inside our human body, it's very easy for cancerous antigens to take over our healthy cells and lead to disease. I think this is the best way I can simplify this for you. if you eat meat, sugar, or lots of processed foods, you are a pretty good candidate for disease showing up in many aspects of your life. Again, I don't wish this on you. Having said that, I can't be there to tell you what to eat all the time either.

Chemicals, additives, and preservatives are laced in our everyday food supply. These are also considered extremely acidic! Take a look at the back of any package you put in your shopping cart at the supermarket. I want you to look for certain things. Just to name a few, there are chemicals that are especially deadly to brain cells. Carrageenan is one of the worst, which in lab studies, has shown to manifest brain tumors. MSG (monosodium glutamate) is another chemical associated with brain tumors, body-wide tumors, and addiction. In an attempt to mask MSG in processed foods, the food industry has given MSG over 40 different names so we cannot recognize it. Talk about 'scumbaggery"!

Let me put forward a point that you all may not have thought about up until now. Migraine headaches are very common, however, they are not normal. You see, I have not had a migraine headache (or a headache of any kind) for 2 years now. Believe me, I don't give you this information to rub it in. The only reason I tell you this is to let you know there are people out there who do not suffer from every day or chronic headaches. Let alone migraine headaches!

Hopefully, I've given you some things to think about in order to give yourselves some relief. There's nothing worse than having one of the most important organs in your body inflamed and giving you issues. Some of you are "Weekday Warriors", dealing with migraine headaches on top of an already increasing workload and family life that may be crippling you mentally! Throwing migraine headaches into that mix is like adding kerosene to an already out-of-control fire.

If you are up for getting rid of your migraine headaches, or any headache, without the use of medications of any kind, then take a look at my video on how to get rid of migraine headaches on my YouTube channel. There are also some rather colorful ways to get rid of a headache in this video! I'll let you watch the video to find out what they are. Here is the link…

https://www.youtube.com/watch?v=vfS3HcVG3I0

I wish you all could click on that instead of reading it! *LOL*

According to the American Chiropractic Association (along with Dr. John Bergman), 97% of all headaches originate in the neck due to compressed nerves and/or forward head carriage (Your head being "set" forward out of alignment with the rest of your cervical spine). Interesting, huh?!

That's all I have for you in this chapter. I'll see you in the next one where we are going to be talking about a woman's issue, namely, menopause!

Section Three

Do You Suffer From Any Of These?

Secret #11: Menopause

Hey Ladies! Yes, I'm talking to all you of you out there complaining right now of those HOT FLASHES. Yes, you! I don't know why I started this paragraph off with "Hey Ladies", but I was a Beastie Boys fan back in the day, so that might have a little bit to do with it. Enough with my musical history lesson, it's time to tell you all what you want to know about menopause and how to get control of this mid-life beast!

What is menopause anyway? Well, I've found the best definition for any type of medical disease is a simple one. Menopause is the end of your child bearing days! This is your body's way of saying "I quit"! No more buying little cute blue or pink outfits. No more little booties that immediately flush your face with excitement and instantly turns you giddy with childlike awe. No more cute, little fat cheeks to squeeze. Best of all, no more poopy diapers or urine fountains! Yeah, I know you don't' miss that last one. *LOL*

In addition, you won't be having any more monthly visitors. Aunt Flo has taken her last rest stop at your place. Now, I know some of you NEVER want to see your monthly visitor again! No more tampons! Some of you have this date marked on your calendar but there are some serious consequences to not having your monthly menstrual cycle. Let's talk about some of these consequences in-depth now, as they may shed some light on recent health problems you might have been experiencing, but not knowing exactly where they were originating from.

Hot Flashes. My wife literally calls these "Hell on Earth!" They interrupt sleep, cause <u>dehydration</u>, and result in "the chills" from excess sweating. So how do we stop this devilish attack on a woman's body? We must take care of the body as a whole, then the body takes care of itself. Treating only the affected area is an exercise in futility.

The overriding structure causing hot flashes is in the regulatory part of the brain, known as the hypothalamus. This part close to the midbrain actually regulates body temperature. In my research for this book, many textbooks and websites reference an imbalance in estrogen as being the cause for the dysfunction of the hypothalamus. This information is dead wrong! If you know anything about the physiology of the body, the hypothalamus actually controls the pituitary gland, the master gland. The pituitary gland controls all the other glands. If a secretion from one of the secondary glands is able to affect the hypothalamus, then the hypothalamus actually would have no control at all.

Thus, there has to be another reason why the hypothalamus is allowing a fluctuation in your body temperature. I believe the deviation in body temperature from one extreme to the other is due to impurities in the tissues of the brain, not just the hypothalamus. Every woman goes through menopause, so I can't say that it's a tumor or a lesion on the hypothalamus that's causing this issue. However, from observations and case studies, I do know that most American women do eat a western diet filled with chemicals, additives, and preservatives.

It is my opinion that the toxification of the hypothalamus and the pituitary gland are the main culprits for extreme body temperature fluctuations. We are vehemently bombarded every single day with toxins affecting our brain tissue. Just a few examples are vaccines, polluted air, fluoridated and chlorinated water, and preservatives used in packaged foods. This infection of our brain by everyday adjuvants can lead to the next item featured on this list.

Memory Loss. My everyday occupation is an anatomy and physiology instructor at a medical college. Most of the faculty and staff working there are women of varying ages. Some of these women are approaching menopause or in full-on menopausal transition. It's not a pretty sight to see one of your fellow co-workers walking up the hall trying to give a tour when she's sweating like a football quarterback after his offensive lineman missed an assignment!

Concurrently, the same antigens responsible for the damage of the hypothalamus, are the same antigens that will rob you of your memory. Memory is often controlled by the hippocampus. This is another part of the brain easily infected by erroneous adjuvants. Long term memory is often left unaffected, however, short-term memory is very sporadic at best. Now don't get me wrong, just because you've looked around your house for 5 minutes in an attempt to find your glasses only to find they were on your face, does not mean you have menopause! *LOL*

On the flip side though, if you find yourself unable to finish sentences over the course of the past few months or recall the most basic of information that you could easily muster in previous years, there may be cause for concern IF you are going through menopause. Just to be clear, brain games on your smartphone will not fix this!

Decrease In Reproductive Hormones. Women tend to know a lot about their bodies, as they go to the doctor a lot more often than men. Most women can tell you the two main hormones responsible for reproduction in their bodies. If you haven't guessed by now, they are estrogen and progesterone. Estrogen is responsible for a woman's secondary sex characteristics. Progesterone is a powerful chemical secreted by the corpus luteum to maintain a woman's fetus for the first three months of pregnancy.

Like I said before, some of you are looking forward to this change. I can't blame you, bloodletting every month can cause extreme fatigue. I have to ask a serious question now though: Have you ever thought about what happens when these two major female hormones disappear? Let's list a few...

Sagging Skin
Thin Lips
Excessive Body Hair
Painful Intercourse
Vaginal Dryness
Thin Body Skin
Visible (Varicose) Veins
Weight Gain
Dehydration
...And More...(I know this sounds like an infomercial but it's accurate!)

You see, it sounds a lot better than it is. You may want menopause to come as soon as possible, but what you're wishing on yourself is far worse health wise! Don't cut off your nose to spite your face. Some of you may not know that phrase, so let me put it another way... Don't shorten your life for convenience!

Irregular Heartbeat. In my opinion, this is the scariest of the symptoms from menopause. When our heart malfunctions, it feels like the end of our life is near. No one, and I mean no one, likes that feeling! Combined that with some of the other symptoms and you might just think that you're dying!

Here is what you may find puzzling. After you've had an episode of palpitations and a possible irregularity in your heartbeat, you may head to the doctor to try to find out what's going on. Usually when women go to have these cardiac assessments done, nothing is found to be wrong with their hearts! So what's causing all of the irregular activity that's making you nervous? It's called hypomineralization.

In today's society, we don't get anywhere near the nutrients required by our body to function properly. In truth, we hardly get any. This is why most holistic and naturopathic doctors of today recommend supplementation along with a plant-based diet. That way, we can cover all the bases. Just to get a little bit more specific for you, the main supplements needed to maintain a supremely healthy heart and valves include niacin, copper, and vanadium. Don't get me wrong, I don't want you to stop there. These are just heart-specific.

Note: Niacin is hard on our livers. It should only be taken...
#Once every 3 days (if you are exhibiting heart disease symptoms).
#Once per week (if you are using this to prevent heart disease).

An irregular heartbeat will lead to skips in blood supply, which can cause anemia. Anemia is usually indicated by our extremities becoming very cold very fast. In addition to this, we can also have air bubbles floating through arteries and veins which can cause problems all their own. We can't have lapses in pressure in a pressure system, as vital organs will be severely damaged or even fail!

Underactive Thyroid. This condition is also known as hypothyroidism. Our thyroid gland is responsible for our metabolism. Metabolism is defined as the amount of work your bodily cells do in performing their functions. This "work" performed by our cells actually dictates how fast we lose fat and how much fat we lose.

This state of low activity from our thyroid gland will actually lead to effortless weight gain. Since this is one biological function most humans would rather not have, I should probably tell you what's causing this problem. Chemical and physical stress are two of the main culprits here. Stress is the overriding factor when it comes to an under-producing thyroid.

Cortisol is the stress hormone that efficiently destroys inflammation within our bodies. When in short supply, cortisol must steal to remain active. Thus, it will "borrow" precursors from other parts of the body in order to produce more cortisol. Those precursors usually come from your thyroid gland first. This results in a thyroid that is larger in size but less efficient in function. This can trigger an enormous weight gain for no apparent reason! This will also trigger Chronic Fatigue Syndrome, meaning you are tired most of the time, no matter what time of day it is.

Insomnia. Having trouble sleeping is a problem for most of us nowadays. For some reason, we can't get a good night's sleep due to excessive media devices delivering all types of invasive, disruptive messages right before we go to bed. When our brain's rhythms are disrupted, it's very hard to get any type of sleep, let alone, good sleep. So let's find out why you're not sleeping well.

There are two glands in the brain that start with the letter "P". One we've already mentioned called the pituitary gland. However, most people do not know of the other "P" gland we called the pineal gland. The pineal gland secretes a hormone called melatonin, which rushes into our bloodstream in dimly lit rooms or at our designated bedtime. Usually, we have trained this gland to secrete at a specific time during the evening, that's the time when you get sleepy.

Well, according to the latest studies, most Americans' pineal glands are calcified. This means the gland is hardened and unable to perform its function optimally, if at all. If you start taking sleeping pills to placate yourself, you are ultimately shutting down your pineal gland! Our brains make decisions by the nanosecond. The minute your brain determines that a substance is coming from outside your body to carry out a function, it will cease to produce that same chemical inside your body. Thus, you become dependent on higher and higher doses of the external chemical to enable you to get good sleep.

Add menopause to this already widespread epidemic and you can see why menopausal women are capping out at two hours sleep per night...maximum! This decrease in hormones secreted by the brain, including the pituitary gland, means less electrical activity in the uterus and ovaries. Less electrical activity means less hormone production. Less hormone production means less physiological activity, and less physiological activity results in the problems we are talking about in this very chapter.

The Fix. You might be asking, "How do I fix this?" Eating a **plant-based diet** every day is the best way I know to avoid all these problems. In fact, you can go from a postmenopausal state to a pre-menopausal state just by making this simple change.

I also recommend hyper-mineralization. Our food supply of late is devoid of any nutrients our body needs to keep itself going. One vitamin I highly recommend is **Andrew Lessman's Essential 1 Multivitamin**. It comes very close to satisfying all the nutritional needs we require on a daily basis. Another one I've found that's been excellent is **Organic Liquid Nighttime Multi-Mineral by Mary Ruth**. Using these two together should give you most of your essential vitamins and minerals. After a few weeks following this protocol, you'll be waving bye-bye to your menopausal status!

A few key nutrients needed to reverse your menopause and alleviate the former conditions are amino acids (key), acetyl-L-carnitine, Gingko, and magnesium. Why?

Well, the **magnesium** helps with normal digestive function and delivering nutrients to the reproductive organs for proper function. This will also help manage any heart issues displayed during menopause.

Ginkgo extract will help return those sexual "juices" back to their past glory! Sound good?! I thought you might like that. That's another way of saying it preserves the firmness of your vaginal walls and maintains the function of your Bartholin glands.

Acetyl-L-carnitine helps manage weigh gain, so you don't blow up like a balloon when it's time for your period to die! It's widely known that women have a hard time losing weight during menopause. This significant hormone stops this.

Amino acids are necessary for the reverse of menopause and the return of normalized function of the reproductive system. These amino acid supplements will also support all of the above nutrients to incorporate properly for optimal function.

OoooooWee! That was a long one, but no harm done. Only health. So, I'll see you in the next chapter.

Section Three

Do You Suffer From Any Of These?

Secret #12: Depression

I know there are entire series of texts on the subject of depression, so I won't pretend this is an exhaustive explanation or remedy for the condition. I do believe I've found some key points that will help anybody who is suffering with depression right now...without the need for destructive medications. My solution to your depression involves more than just a change in diet, as that was all that was needed in dealing with other conditions in this book. Depression though, is a little bit more complicated. We will go a little bit deeper in this chapter and finding out how to truly help you get rid of your depression.

Let's start with a more obvious things. Just because you have a bad day, a bad week, or a bad month, don't believe you are now entering the world of depression. Everyone has bad days or even bad extended periods of time. What I'm about to say next is all important when dealing with your condition effectively. Never, and I mean never, compare your mental situation with that of another person! Your body chemistry, blood composition, physiological set-points, and hormone distribution is unique to you. What works for others, won't necessarily work for you. So stop comparing!

On this situation, you cannot be a follower. If you sincerely want to get rid of this horrid condition that has shortened many lives on this Earth, then you'll have to take the lead in conquering your depression. Most people who deal with this believe depression is purely psychological. This couldn't be any further from the truth. Any time a human being generates a "feeling", that "feeling" is brought about by a chemical secreted into the bloodstream! I bet you didn't know that your happiness came from your own personal, internal pharmacy...better known as serotonin and dopamine.

It's time to get real here! Drugs like Zoloft, Prozac, Celexa, and Paxil are effective for a brief period, but after about two months, the depression comes back with a vengeance! Why? You really didn't deal with the problem, just tried to mask the symptoms, and even that's not working. This class of drugs are known as SSRIs (selective-serotonin reuptake inhibitors). SSRIs block the reabsorption of serotonin for the purpose of making more available after the drug wears off. This has a temporary mood-boosting on the individual. However, the drug will wear off! Your depression is right back "center-stage" and sometimes worse than your previous episodes.

Ah, I can hear your wheels turning inside that head of yours! You are thinking to yourself, "Well, I'll just keep on taking the pills". Whoa, whoa Gingah! Hasn't anybody told you to read the package insert, especially to see what kind of side effects could happen from prolonged use of these drugs? If not, I'm telling you now. Of all the side effects listed for these nefarious drugs, one stands out more than any other: DEPRESSION! Huh! Wait, anti-depression medication causes depression?! You got it, Slim.

How can they get away with this?! Let's see, pharmaceutical companies have no legal liability for any injury (National Childhood Vaccine Injury Act (NCVIA) of 1986 (42 U.S.C. §§ 300aa-1 to 300aa-34)), no matter how severe. You don't even get to go to trial for damage done to you or your family members for any reason. You will have to attend an arbitration meeting called "Vaccine Court". Just one more way to circumvent your rights! "Vaccine court" is a convincing circus meant to look official, so as to make you believe it's official. In truth, it's nothing but the pharmaceutical companies *playing* "court" and pretending justice is being served.

I don't expect you to simply believe what I say or write, so I'll just show you what I found:

[Drugs.com]

- darkened urine
- decreased urine output
- decreased vision
- depressed mood
- difficulty with breathing
- difficulty with speaking
- difficulty with swallowing
- drooling
- dry skin and hair
- eye pain

I just want to check to see if you're looking at the exact same thing that I'm looking at. To your left and four bullet points down, I have listed one of the "rare" side effects of Zoloft. A drug that claims it can treat depression should not cause a "depressed mood".

By the way, that's pharmaceutical speak for depression!

Keep in mind, this is only ten of over a hundred side effects present with this particular drug. If an individual were taking a combination of drugs for depression, the list of side effects could easily equal 250 or more! Being that this is so scary, I'm going to have you all do a bit of homework right now. Don't worry, it's pretty easy. All you have to do is take out your smartphone right now, go to YouTube.com, then search "Latuda TV commercial". This commercial lists some of the worst symptoms I've ever heard for any medication for any condition. They don't even wait till the end to start telling you it can possibly kill you!

I have to point out something here, there is a big difference between clinically diagnosed depression and being discouraged (feeling down). Everyone feels discourage at some point in their life. This is nothing new and should not be confused with depression of any kind. As stated earlier though, most depression can be traced back to a chemical imbalance of serotonin in the brain. Let me take this a step further, depression not only affects your mental state, but also your physiology in all parts of your body. Muscles, soft tissues, and nerve cells are also affected, leading me to believe that dopamine (another neurotransmitter in the brain) is also affected.

Lack of dopamine is what causes tremors in Parkinson's disease. Since one of the main symptoms of using SSRIs is uncoordinated gait (unable to walk properly), I have to believe that dopamine is also being affected by the use of these prescribed depression medications. Remember, these are only my opinions and should not be mistaken for medical advice. I do, however, believe in my assessment tremendously! I have helped people get over depression in a relatively short period of time (as little as two months) and have proven to myself and my clients, my methods work better than any destructive pills!

Now that you've heard the Bad and the Ugly, let's get to the Good. Most medical books and websites are going to tell you depression is easily treatable. I tend to agree with them, but for different reasons. These online and medical publications believe pharmaceutical drugs are the answer. Needless to say, I don't! My question is, why would you take something for the rest of your life that could possibly be harmful and increase the intensity of the very condition you are trying to get rid of? I know, some of us just want to get the pain gone! Nonetheless, in the long run, it's not worth it.

I have a very different take on treating depression. Pharmaceutical drugs for depression are destructive at best. Thus, I will never recommend them for the treatment of any condition, let alone depression. Fruits and vegetables were put here for a reason. I believe their purpose is to nourish us with the necessary nutrients and vitamins we need. Unfortunately, over time our industrialized nations have turned gathering food into an assembly line instead of a garden. I believe there is a serious link between eating our necessary fruits and vegetables and outstanding mental health.

Here are some things you can do research on right now and conclude for yourself how important food is to excellent mental status. All you have to do is look, the information is out there!

≡ TIME | Health

DIET/NUTRITION

The Strange Link Between Junk Food and Depression

Mandy Oaklander
Jun 29, 2015

Of our many modern diseases, one of the biggest burdens on society is an unexpected one: depression, according to the World Health Organization. And what we eat may be contributing, finds a new study published in the *American Journal of Clinical Nutrition.*

James E. Gangwisch, PhD, assistant professor at Columbia University in the department of psychiatry, wanted to find out whether foods with a higher glycemic index (GI)—a scale that ranks carbohydrate-containing foods by how much they raise your blood sugar—would be associated with greater odds of depression. "When I was a kid, I was almost like a candy junkie," Gangwisch says. "I noticed for myself, if I eat a lot of sugar, it makes me feel down the next day." Gangwisch says he stopped eating added sugar years ago but remained curious about whether a junk food diet could make people depressed.

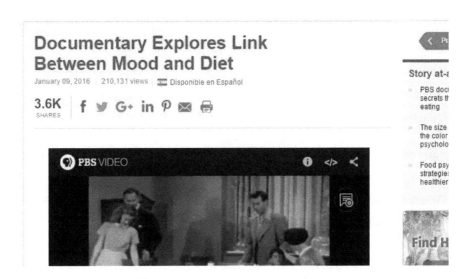

There are hundreds of headlines and new studies just like the ones above. Big Pharma can try all they want to try and conceal the truth. However, there is no hiding from people wanting to get better and doing their own research to find out what can work for them. This is not a game! People are committing suicide at abnormal rates simply because they've been diagnosed with clinical depression and put on these addictive and useless protocols.

Alvin's Protocol For Depression

*** I am not a doctor, nor do I give medical advice. Any and all information is for entertainment purposes. If you wish to try any protocol put forth in this text or via my website, please talk to a doctor first. All information should be taken seriously and given adequate thought as to its use.*

Now that we've got that s**t is out of the way, let's get to transforming your body into a depression-killing, high performance engine! First of all, if you want anything to work, it must be able to be absorbed into the digestive tract. Without doing this step first, you won't hardly notice any change at all. On the other hand, if you do this first step and then take pharmaceutical drugs to treat your depression, this might make your condition a lot worse. I have to warn again, stay away from depression medications!

Step #1. The initial step in making any treatment with depression work is to thoroughly cleanse the colon. There is no use in sending nutrients or minerals of any kind through your digestive system if it's unable to absorb them. So the first step is 2 purify our colon. This will be accomplished using a **saline wash**. All the details for this can be found in my YouTube video called 'How To Do a Colonic - Saline Wash At Home'. Step 1...CHECK!

Before we move on, I should tell you this step alone will help get rid of 75% of your bouts of depression. How could that possibly be? Well, most people don't realize that only 10% of serotonin is produced in the brain. The other 90% of our "happy hormone" is produced in the digestive tract. This is another reason why you should always watch what you're putting into your mouth!

The digestive system is not just a tube you shove food into. It's actually a filtering system that allows you to take nutrients and distribute them to your vital organs WITHOUT delivering toxins at the same time. Talk about an amazing body system! With regard to humans, it seems that someone has thought of everything. One of the amazing facts about this information is, in recent studies done by Oxford University (2002 study), incidences of violence decreased by 34% to 37% in a prison population simply by changing their diet! This is an astounding figure.

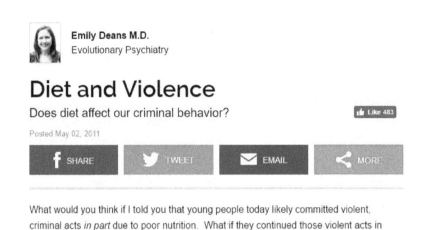

Emily Deans M.D.
Evolutionary Psychiatry

Diet and Violence

Does diet affect our criminal behavior?

Posted May 02, 2011

SHARE   TWEET   EMAIL   MORE

What would you think if I told you that young people today likely committed violent, criminal acts *in part* due to poor nutrition. What if they continued those violent acts in prison as the poor nutrition continued? Reserve judgment for now. This is science - let's

Step #2. Like I always tell my students, "Fruits and vegetables, vitamins and minerals!" You should know by now (from me yapping away in my videos), fruits and vegetables should always be organic. Organic produce is the number one way to get our nutrients to nourish our bodies. Some of the most effective body-healers are leafy green vegetables. Both cilantro and parsley are extremely powerful blood-cleaners. Believe it or not, they help a good deal with depression. This is only one of the many reasons we must ingest fresh organic fruits and vegetables. You can get creative and use whatever you'd like from the vast variety of colorful choices we can eat. Just to get you started, this is what I have every morning without fail.

Alvin J's Own Ultimate Health Food Smoothie:

Carrot (1 whole carrot)
Ginger root (Small piece of a branch)
Beet (¼ of a beet)
Grapefruit (½ a grapefruit)
Spinach (1 handful)
Apple (½ an apple)
Pineapple [optional] (1/4 cup pineapple for sweetness)
Tomato (½ a tomato)
Lemon (½ a lemon)
Supplements (break open the capsule(s) and shake in)

***Mix all of the above together in a NutriBullet/Ninja/Whatever, then drink! I do this every morning, but I'm a nutjob. Please feel free to change up your fruits and veggies weekly to stay excited about doing it. You can add more or less of any of these ingredients for taste or the size of your blending container. I have the NutriBullet Rx.*

Recently, I've been using two super mineralization supplements. Don't forget, our food is woefully devoid of nutrients and minerals. That's why we need the additional supplementation to make up for the gaps in our electrolyte intake. The two super food minerals I've found are called **Andrew Lessman's Essential 1 Multivitamin** and **Organic Liquid Nighttime Multi-Mineral by Mary Ruth**. You can find these links on the right side of my website (HumanHealthLink.com). I mentioned these in a previous chapter, and why shouldn't I? These are two of the most powerful mineralization methods I've utilized to date.

Step #3. Loneliness is the enemy! The reason most people who suffer with depression have their condition worsened, is because they spend inordinate amounts of time alone. We have a funny habit here in the United States with our fast-paced, microwave culture (and I use that term loosely). We tend to overuse our brains, one part in particular. That part of the brain resides right behind that big ole forehead of yours. It's your cortex, or to be more specific, your prefrontal cortex.

This amazing part of your brain allows you to visualize scenarios into the future. Whenever you hear an athlete saying they visualize their performance before they hit the field, they are basically saying they have created a future picture in their mind of what they want to achieve. Contrary to popular belief, this works extraordinarily well! The ability of your mind to create a successful destiny without ever having it happen in real life, is so fascinating it defies explanation.

Our brains have no idea what is real and what is imagined. When I say that, some of you may find that very, very, very hard to believe. I don't blame you for having doubts, so here are some examples you may be able to identify with to solidify this point. Have you ever had a "wet" dream? You know, naked bodies grinding, sweating, and writhing in pure erotic ecstasy! Sounds dirty, right?! The catch is YOU ARE DREAMING.

Now, even though no other person was present in your bedroom, no physical contact took place, and you've gone without getting laid for the last 14 months, somehow you were able to soak your bed sheets with warm sweat, elevate your blood pressure, you are breathing like a maniac, and achieved the best orgasm you've had in 5 years! How can you explain that? Quoting one of the most famous lines in 'The Matrix', "...your brain makes it real".

I layout the previous example to say the following, this is all created by our prefrontal cortex. If you allow your mind to run rampant based off today's societal norms, it will ultimately go to the worst case scenario. This series of mental events is all too common in today's society. If your brain activity is considered normal, you can snap out of this pretty easily. However, if you suffer from depression, this focus on worst-case thinking can end up worsening your depression, building a prison in your mind, and allowing your negative thoughts to ultimately force you to contemplate suicide!

The key here is not to remain alone. New ideas and talking to other human beings, no matter what you are talking about, is one of the best ways to escape your present train of thought. I've also noticed **music** can almost instantly change the pattern of a human being's thought. It doesn't work in every case but music can often yank you out of a funk that might otherwise turn into something horrible. Along the same lines, you may want to change the people you hang around. Friends who don't back you up or don't have your beliefs in common will often sabotage your attempts to be a more positive and productive person. It's all important to free your mind and keep it out of the field of negativity.

I'm sorry about that. I had to get a little deep on you in that last paragraph but you have to realize the people you hang around will ultimately determine your future.

If you don't believe that, I need you to gather your own investigative proof. How about this, go down to your nearest neighborhood projects (the hood) and notice the kind of people that hang together. I'm pretty sure you'll see some iteration of crabs in a barrel! Then I'd like you to go down to a country club or luxury, premium spa. Look around, you might notice the people are very friendly towards each other and even help each other complete business deals and life decisions. I'm not saying that your life will reflect this. I am saying that you should notice the difference between to stark extremes and maybe tailor your life to be more like the latter.

That's all I have for this chapter. If you have any other questions, I will be making a video soon with regard to depression. If you have any more questions, I will be happy to answer your questions in the comments of that video or on my website.

On to the next chapter!

Section Three

Do You Suffer From Any Of These?

Secret #13: A Few Extra Pounds

Have you put on a few extra pounds you want to get rid of...right now? You know what I'm talking about, those cute, creative names we have for our fat...blubber, lard, meaty, thick, chunky, hefty, inflatable, stout, hefty, pudgy, husky, plump, tons of fun, heavy-set, butterball, oversized, big, and my personal favorite...more cushion for the pushin'! Where the f*** did that last one come from?! Obviously, some dude got tired of pushing all that extra out of the way in the midst of his midnight romp to Blubber Town! *LOL*

I'm in a good mood, so let's have some fun with fat. You may have heard of a show that debuted in 2006 called 'Yo Momma'. The host of the show was Wilmer Valderrama and the entire premise of the show was contestants facing off to see who had the best "yo momma" jokes. Here are a few I thought were pretty good…

"Yo momma so fat, when she tried out for a weight loss show, they told her, "Sorry, no groups!""

"Yo momma so fat, when God said, "Let there be light", he leaned over to yo momma and whispered "Move out of the way!""

"Yo momma so fat, she left the house in high heels and came back in flip-flops!"

Ok, ok. I'm done. *LMAO*! Wait, wait one more..."yo momma so fat, Dracula bit her and got diabetes!" *I'm literally having too much fun right now!

Seriously, I don't want to come off as insensitive, so that's the end of the little joke session. It always helps to have a sense of humor when you're dealing with anything you want to improve with your body. I found that laughing is one of the best ways to lose weight and improve your mental state of being. If you don't believe this, then you haven't lived...in my opinion!

First. Let's get to the good stuff. My number one tip for weight loss is to **supply your body with protein** as soon as you wake up in the morning. This tip alone will promote you losing 10 pounds within the next two weeks, if you stick with it. You can get protein in many different forms. So I don't want you to immediately go to the whey protein or muscle-builders for this nutrient. There are plenty of organic alternatives that will supply the same amount of protein as these artificial synthetics.

Some of the more practical foods used to build protein in our bodies include beans, leafy green vegetables, mushrooms, potatoes, sweet corn, and eggs. If you want to go the route of taking a supplement or powder, the best one I found so far is MRM Plant Protein. It blends very well and does not have the awful taste of some of the others I've tried. It is also no secret our bodies manufacture proteins in order to maintain our everyday body processes. As we sleep, however, these stores of protein are then used to rebuild. Therefore, we have to replenish these proteins to continue our daily physiological functions and store those proteins for the next day.

Second. The next action I have for you is what I've been talking about all along. We have to intake fresh, organic fruits and vegetables along with powerful vitamins and minerals to maintain a healthy lifestyle. I know I've said that time and time again, but the only way I think you'll take this information seriously is to beat it into you until you can't forget it! One more time: Fruits and vegetables, vitamins and minerals!

Third. Next, we have to eliminate all processed and white foods from our diet if you really want to get serious about weight loss. Think of the food you eat when I refer to "white foods". Sugar, flour, bread, pasta, Etc. These foods ultimately have one thing in common, they turn into sugar when eaten. Barring any extreme physical fitness, our bodies don't require much sugar at all. Our main energy source has been converted to sugar via our unsanitary, chemical-laden diet. Our real source of energy should be fat!

In science or history class, you may have heard of a phenomenon called the "hunter-gatherer days". What that meant was a human being would hunt for their food, eat as much of that food as possible, then go for long periods of time without eating because hunting wasn't always easy. During those lean times of famine, we would have to rely on our built up fat stores from our binging on hunted meals previously. Fat, for a human being, is the most optimum form of energy production. The storage of fat implies that one day your body will use it. Unfortunately, there are restaurants on every corner, 30 coffee shops in every neighborhood, and everyone loves to use alcohol as their favorite fun pastime.

The inclusion of these unsafe staples in our everyday diet is not something we can sustain long-term. We all have different ideas for what is good and bad for our bodies, mainly from watching TV commercials and watching news stories. There are so many news stories and articles online telling us what to eat and what not to eat. It's absolutely confusing and frustrating at the same time! Here are some things I've found to be true from my own personal experience. Let's see if you can pick up a pattern here…

Hamburgers…BAD
Bacon…GOOD
American cheese…BAD
Organic hand-made cheese…GOOD
Pizza Hut…BAD
Artisan brick-oven pizza…GOOD
Ice cream…BAD
Hand-made ice cream…GOOD
Beer…BAD
Eggs…GOOD
Country Crock spread…BAD
100% Butter…GOOD
Birthday cake…BAD
Fruits and veggies/vitamins and minerals…AMAZING!

I think you kinda get the hint. I'm a little bit of a weirdo when it comes to eating food. Here's what I mean, I always pay attention to how I feel after I eat anything. Do I feel light-headed? Do I have an upset stomach? Did my mood change unnecessarily when I was happy before? Do I have a headache now? You should always pay attention to how your body feels after you eat a certain food. If you notice feelings that most would consider negative AFTER eating, then it's a safe assumption THAT food is not working for you. Never mind what anybody else says is healthy or unhealthy, the brief suggestions I gave you above on what's good and bad are from my personal experience. Some of the foods I've listed as "bad" might work for you and some I've listed as "good" may NOT work for you.

Fourth. The last action I have for you, as far as losing weight, is a whole body cleanse. Usually when we talked about cleanses, most of you will have an image of a colonic. A colonic cleanse (or digestive flush) is just one of the avenues we have to cover when losing weight. The two other major paths for losing weight are even more important, those being cleansing the tissues and cleansing the liver. I will go much more in-depth about the liver in chapter 15, but for right now, I'll give you the shiny nuggets to keep those extra pounds off.

At one time or another in our lives, we've all been susceptible to the lure of the infomercial. They show you ripped, sweaty, fitness models that have the very body that you ache for! The only problem is... you have to buy this product within the next 30 minutes in order to get that dream body you want. In the commercial, they make it appear as if no work is required. All you have to do is buy this magical program and all of your problems will be solved. At some time during this psychological mind f***, you suspend your disbelief just long enough to jump online and order the product that you think will bring you the body of a lifetime. What happens next is what pisses you off! You get the program, open the box, put it on your favorite shelf, and swear to yourself you're going to get to using this on the first free Monday you get. *We always want to start at the beginning of the week, so we can eat like a starving hog on that weekend...*LOL* You aint slick!*

Both you and I know the minute you put that product on the shelf, is the moment you decided that you were never going to use it. Fitness programs are not the only thing that's getting money out of you with no return on your bodily investment. Diet pills, organic packaged foods, meals to your front door, and insane television commercial promises are all part of the advertising mix to get you to buy the next thing you'll never use. Think about that, billions of dollars are spent on all of these gimmicks and promotions only to find out Americans are the most overweight population on the planet! If we spend the most money on health and wellness, then how are we the fattest nation in existence? That doesn't make sense does it? Well, it doesn't make since to me either.

Now I'm going to assume you are not one of the average, run-of-the-mill slackers mentioned in the paragraph above. I know if you bought a program, you would at least use it, and hopefully, stick with it. Let's assume that you even got great results out of using one of these programs and/or pills. There's always a slowdown phase in any weight loss called a plateau.

This phase is often hit while you are about 75% of the way to your weight loss goal. You started off at 250 pounds, then you got down to 220 pounds, next stop 190 pounds, then you get all the way down to 175 pounds. What you've done so far is no small feat! Congratulations! This is awesome and you are ecstatic about your hard work, your final goal wasn't 175 lbs. though. It was 130lbs.

Something strange happened. Now, you work out for another month only to find that you are still 175 pounds. So you work out another month, and still no change. You worked out for another 2 months consecutively doing everything that you did to get down to your 175-pound status, but the pounds are no longer coming off. What in the hell is going on?! The answer: POISON.

Our fat cells are absolutely necessary for our physiological well-being. However, they have one overriding flaw that can bring down the entire system...they store poisons! The foods we eat in a modern diet have hardly any nutrients at all but are packed with additives, preservatives, and chemicals. For most of these adjuvants found in our food supply, our body has no idea how to biologically process them. Since this is the case, these foreign bodies cannot be allowed to float around in our blood, as this would cause toxicity of the blood.

There are two places that commonly accumulate these excess cytotoxins...our joint and our fat cells. Joints have wide open spaces and are encased in a bursa sac. This is an ideal place to store antigens, due to lack of blood interaction and a large lumen (opening).

In addition to this, our fat cells commonly accept trash through their walls in a martyr-like fashion to protect our blood supply. If you bring "junk" to a nervous cell, it will say, "No, no! Take that crap down the hall!" Similarly, if you take the same "junk" to a muscle cell, it will do the exact same thing. The only cell in your body that accepts non-essential debris is your fat cells. When you bring "junk" to a fat cell it says, "Ok...um...put it over there in that corner".

This is where the problem lies. The accumulation of these poisons in our fat cells is protecting our blood supply from harm. If your body allows you to burn these infected fat cells, then the poison will be released into your blood. Your body will make every effort not to poison itself, thus, it will prevent you from burning these fat cells for energy. We talked about a plateau a few minutes ago, where you are unable to lose any more weight. Well, this is the very cause of that phenomenon. Since your body makes it almost impossible to burn these fat cells, we have to use more concentrated, external methods to make this happen.

Enter the Gaia Supreme Cleanse. I've tried about 10 cleanses now, and the Gaia Supreme Cleanse is the best one I've found so far. First, it is not a laxative like many others on the market. Next, it does not promote stomach issues and abdominal cramping either. The very best thing about this particular cleanse is there is no need to hang around a toilet for fear of explosive diarrhea! It just works with your natural bowel movement. Having said that, if you are going to buy anything, I would put my money on this one.

Thyroid Issues. The thyroid gland, found on the front of our voice box, is the gland responsible for our metabolism. Most people in today's society have either hyperthyroidism or hypothyroidism, meaning an overproducing thyroid or an under-producing thyroid. If you have an overproducing thyroid, you can pretty much eat whatever you'd like and never gain a pound! I know that might sound like the best thing ever, but that does not mean your arteries are not clogged or that you are free of disease. On the flip side, if you have an under-producing thyroid, if you sniff a grape, you'll gain 10 pounds! That may be a little bit of an exaggeration, but I want you all to get the point.

Hyperthyroidism is usually caused by an overproduction by the thyroid due to a tumor being present or a lack of secretion by the parathyroid glands themselves. In either case, this causes the thyroid gland to over secrete T3 and T4. We have glands on the back of the thyroid called parathyroid glands that help balance the frequency of metabolic work. It's supposed to be a partnership to keep everything in balance.

Because cells do their work according to how hormones are released from the pituitary gland, we must keep the hypothalamus, controller of the pituitary gland, healthy. This can be done by the very diet we've mentioned earlier in this book. Fruits and vegetables, vitamins and minerals! Without keeping this all-important part of the brain working at optimum, none of the glands of the body will secrete hormones correctly. Blighting our bodies with dietary poison can add to weight gain simply by excess inflammation in infected tissues. Again, diet is paramount!

Hypothyroidism mean metabolism levels are low. Just like it sounds, your cells are not doing the work they are supposed to do at the levels required. This will lead to weight gain via available fat not being used for energy. Eating excessive calories (a high-fat, high sugar diet) on a daily basis makes this process even worse, leading to even more added pounds. Just because the thyroid gland slows down production does not mean the parathyroids do the same thing. Underproduction by the thyroid while the parathyroids work at the same output still results in low thyroid production.

Usually, we don't exhibit both of these conditions at the same time. Nevertheless, both cause a significant weight gain that will hinder any weight loss efforts. If you are trying to lose weight, I would definitely suggest you get your thyroid checked to make sure you're not working out for nothing. You may have to go to the doctor so they can give you your readings, however, I am not saying to take anything the doctor gives you.

Let me make myself very clear, you can go to the doctor to get test results to find out blood sugar levels, blood lipid levels, urine analysis, and your metabolic rate. This is the part where you have to listen good! Do not take any medications, any prescriptions, or any advice the doctor gives you that is contradictory to what you've read here. If you have a holistic doctor or a naturopath, they'll probably suggest the exact same things I am suggesting to you now. However, if you participate in traditional medicine, there will always be a protocol for using medications and/or surgery to fix problems.

One of the biggest fears I have for people working towards a healthy lifestyle is the proliferation of weight loss television shows. There is a show called 'The Biggest Loser', and the goal of this show is to lose the most weight among your competitors to win the grand prize. Ultimately, I believe this is a great motivator to get people to lose weight. On the other hand, there always comes a part in the show where the contestants consider a weight loss surgery. They often refer to it as skin removal surgery. Often times, the contestants lose so much weight so quickly, their skin cannot shrink fast enough to accommodate the rapid weight loss. Thus, the need for the surgery.

What they don't tell you: If you lose weight at a reasonable rate about (1 to 2 pounds per week) there is no need to have a skin removal surgery! Well, I think you've heard enough on this issue. I think you get what I'm trying to say about losing weight and how to do it safely.

I'm going to visit you all in the next chapter where we will be a talking about the importance and the DANGERS of hygiene!

Section Three

Do You Suffer From Any Of These?

Secret #14: Brushed Teeth, Fresh Underarms, and Clean Skin...Dangerous?

You all like movies, Right? Well, I would venture to guess that about 25% of movies begin with a sequence of fast-paced millennials getting ready for their morning interaction with the outside world. They are quickly brushing their teeth, soaping up in a hot shower, and slathering deodorant on their shaved underarms. That sounds like the average American morning to me! Before you get too comfortable in recognizing this commonplace routine, you should know...it's killing you!

You might be thinking to yourself, "I can't do anything anymore!" In the traditional sense, you are exactly correct. Let's be honest, nowadays *traditional* will put an end to your life. I'm sure that's not the answer you were looking for when you started reading this book, however, the fact that you ARE reading this book is going to help reverse this trend of early morbidity.

The title to this chapter is quite intriguing, don't you think? I wanted to create some doubt in your fertile mind about your everyday routine. Just because ninety-nine percent of Americans perform the exact same rituals, doesn't mean you should follow suit. The title of this chapter implies that there are dangers lurking in the very things you do every morning to prepare for school or work. This is the magic of the human mind. There is nothing more powerful on this planet than a human being's routine!

Once our brain becomes accustomed to something, our reticular activating system (RAS) kicks in to create a routine that is hardwired into the cerebrum. This routine is created to make your life easier, in effect, ensuring your survival. Our primitive brain is a modern marvel far beyond the understanding of most. Here is where the flaw comes in, our brain can be trained by commercials and modern media. This submission to disruptive brainwashing via television commercials, infomercials, and flashing internet ads has turned us into a nation of rabid consumers. The more sinister motivation behind this: Once a human brain has been trained to do something, it is nearly impossible to break that habit!

I'm going to exaggerate this point just a bit. If you could get "Rachel" (fictional character) to willingly ingest trace amounts of rat poison over the course of 21 days (the time it takes to form a habit), "Rachel" (of her own free-will) will take the rat poison on her own on the 22nd day! Coincidentally, she will take the poison every day after that going forward. I know at the beginning of this paragraph I told you this would be an exaggerated example, I LIED! This is actually happening every day to millions of Americans.

Have you ever heard of Equal, NutraSweet, Saccharin, or Splenda? I'm pretty sure you've heard of at least one of these. What do they all have in common? ASPARTAME! Oh, you don't recognize this deadly chemical by this name. Let me give you one that's more familiar to you. Aspartame is also known as RAT POISON! Do I have your attention now?! Allow me to further blow your mind.

Have you ever thought of shaving calories from your diet by drinking diet colas? This is one of the worst things you could ever do to your body! Diet sodas are only called sugar-free because there's no actual sugar in the drink. However, this diet drink still taste sweet. That's because there is a sugar substitute in your diet cola. You want to take a guess as to what that substitute is? You guessed it, it's aspartame!

Now that you get my drift about how routine and false assumptions can take years, even decades off your life, it's time to get down to the meat of this chapter. I'm going to explain some rather heavy concepts to you about your everyday habits and how you must change them if you want to live your whole life. You might think this is just rhetoric I'm speaking to try to sell this book or to scare you into buying something. Trust me, it is not. The world IS in a profit-driven conspiracy to kill you. Intentional or unintentional, the result is the same...we die!

Brushed Teeth. Public enemy #1 in your medicine cabinet are over the counter and prescribed medications. In a very close second is a substance you never thought was causing harm to your body tissues. That substance is toothpaste. I know this is hard to fathom, but I hear another question rolling around your head again, "Why would they (you mean the FDA) allow a toxic goo to be sold on the open market that causes birth defects, cancer, and brain damage in adults?" The simple answer...because they are paid to.

Like I said, I know this is hard to believe. So don't take my word for it, take a look at some of the information that's out there that you can freely find on your own. Here are some ingredients found in most toothpaste sold over the counter, along with their descriptions.

What	Why you should avoid it
FD & C Color Pigments	Synthetic coloring agents made from coal tar which can be found in a multitude of personal care products, including lip balm/gloss. Known carcinogen.
Propylene Glycol	The EPA considers this ingredient so toxic that for handling, it requires gloves, protective clothing, goggles & disposal by burying.
Parabens	May play a role in sterility in males, hormone imbalances and breast cancer.
Sodium Lauryl/Laureth Sulfate	Has been implicated in oral conditions, including canker sores & bad breath. It's the stuff that makes some toothpaste foamy.
Polyethylene glycol	Linked to production of dangerous levels of dioxin, a cancer causing agent also known to reduce immunity and cause nervous system disorders.
Triclosan	Suspected cancer-causing agent, and connected to hormone imbalances. Has been shown to be toxic to fish and other aquatic animals and plants.

It's amazing when you find out the truth! The phony commercials with teenagers having bright, white smiles by using these "extraordinary, new toothpastes" all turns out to be a bunch of bulls**t! The descriptions given next to these toxic components of toothpaste will seriously degrade any adults health, and let's not talk about the devastating impact it can have on children. If this doesn't bother you, go ahead and keep brushing, tearing open your gums, and introducing acute poisons directly into your bloodstream. Like I said, I am not the government and

I can't force you to do anything. You've been given choice, too bad they are all unhealthy ones.

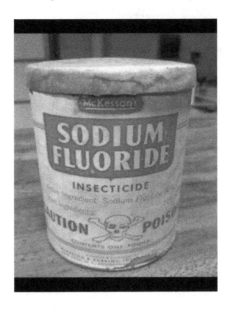

The last time I went to a dentist (about 12 years ago), I was given an interesting option at the end of my dental cleaning. The dentist asked, "Would you like a fluoride treatment?" Being an avid watcher of TV, I believed fluoride was the best thing since Nintendo! So I accepted the fluoride treatment and had my teeth and gums soaked in this modern miracle of dental invention. The blowing of my mind came later when I found out sodium fluoride (above) could maim or even kill me!

Sodium fluoride is the main ingredient in insecticides and pesticides. I didn't know that s***! Did you? Upon further research, I've uncovered this viperous chemical to be a neurological agent, capable of causing brain damage leading to autism, Asperger's, loss of memory, and mental retardation. Here comes the messed up part... they dump copious amounts of this deadly toxin into our water supply! That's in addition to the deadly toothpaste. This is why I said earlier it's almost impossible to escape being poisoned using today's foods apply.

Here is the back of a real tooth paste container, take a look at the warnings and ask yourself why are you putting this in your mouth! Take a look...

Drug Facts	Drug Facts (continued)
Active Ingredient — **Purpose** Sodium monofluorophosphate 0.76% — Anti-Cavity Toothpaste	pea sized amount in children under 6. Supervise children's brushing until good habits are established. Children under **2 yrs.: ask a dentist**
Use: Helps prevent against cavities	**Inactive Ingredients:** Sorbitol, Silica, Water, Sodium Lauryl Sulfate, Flavor, PEG-32, Mica, Sodium Carboxy Methyl Cellulose, Saccharin, Trisodium Phosphate, FD&C Blue No. 1, Calcium Glycerophosphate
Warnings: Keep out of reach of children under 6 years of age. If you accidentally swallow more than used for brushing, get medical help or contact a Poison Control Center immediately.	

It literally says, if swallowed, call Poison Control! Now that you can see how harmful this can actually be to any human being, let me present you with an alternative. First, let me explain. Most Americans only relegate themselves to the options that are available in their closest supermarket. If this is what you limit your options to, you're screwed!

So, what should you use instead of toothpaste? **Baking soda.** I don't even use commercial mouthwash in my morning routine. I've learned the supreme benefits of **hydrogen peroxide** and now use that as a mouthwash. Here's a little trick if you would like to see the foaming effect of toothpaste while using these two super ingredients.

First, gargle for about 30 to 60 seconds with hydrogen peroxide. Then, spit out 75% of the hydrogen peroxide keeping 25% in your mouth. Last, drown your toothbrush in baking soda and brush! This will cause the foaming effect most people like with toothpaste but it has an active whitening effect on your teeth.
Enjoy!

Fresh Underarms. I know some of you have been told that you should never leave the house without putting on deodorant. It is a fact, our bodies stink! After just a little bit of activity, we started sloughing off skin cells, sweating, and secreting from our glands. All this mixed together creates something I like to call STANK!

Whether I'm at the gym, at the grocery store, or at a nice restaurant, I see people smelling themselves. I guess someone wrote in a magazine somewhere that you should be always doing your "smell check" to make sure nobody else can experience your STANK!

Ah, the wonders of curious inventors. The first trademarked deodorant, called 'Mum', debuted in 1888 by an unknown Philadelphia inventor. It was a paste spread under the arms to prevent unwanted odor during the day. Because pastes are not practical, an aerosolized variation appeared soon after.

Today, we use deodorant routinely. We don't even think about it anymore, it's part of your normal morning rituals conditioned into your brain by watching your parents slather it on over and over again. You don't wear deodorant because it keeps you from smelling, you wear deodorant because you've been trained to!

The fragrant scent you experience is just a bonus for your years of dedicated rearing.

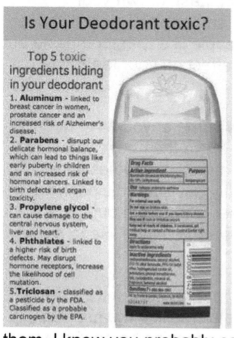

Is Your Deodorant toxic?

Top 5 toxic ingredients hiding in your deodorant

1. **Aluminum** - linked to breast cancer in women, prostate cancer and an increased risk of Alzheimer's disease.
2. **Parabens** - disrupt our delicate hormonal balance, which can lead to things like early puberty in children and an increased risk of hormonal cancers. Linked to birth defects and organ toxicity.
3. **Propylene glycol** - can cause damage to the central nervous system, liver and heart.
4. **Phthalates** - linked to a higher risk of birth defects. May disrupt hormone receptors, increase the likelihood of cell mutation.
5. **Triclosan** - classified as a pesticide by the FDA. Classified as a probable carcinogen by the EPA.

To your left, you will notice a familiar sight. That is a stick of the deodorant, that is more than likely, in your medicine cabinet right now. Right next to this bar of your favorite deodorant is a description of the ingredients. I want you to just look at the list of ingredients, noting there is nothing healthy or natural about any of them. I know you probably can't read the descriptions of these ingredients all that well but I'll spell them out briefly for you.

Once again, you should be asking yourself, "Why would the FDA allow this to happen?" I think you know the answer, so let's move on to some of these noxious ingredients found in your local, neighborhood deodorant. I want you to pay close attention to a couple of things: the ingredients are chemicals and some of the same ingredients were found in your toothpaste! Here's a brief breakdown of the ingredients harmful to us in deodorants...

1. **Aluminum or Aluminum Oxides** - Active metal in antiperspirants which clogs the sweat glands. A 2003 study of 437 women found cancer was diagnosed earlier in women who used

antiperspirants and deodorants. Those who shaved, then used the metal were more likely to develop cancer. Scientists theorized that nicks in the skin allowed the metal to access the bloodstream. It is also estrogen mimicking, leading to cancer.

2. **Parabens** - Used as a preservative. Parabens also mimic estrogen in the body. This leads to a strong possibility of developing cancer in the near future.

3. **Propylene glycol** - A synthetic liquid used to absorb water (sweat) and maintain moisture. The Agency For Toxic Substances And Disease Registry lists it as a potential effector for dermal (skin), renal (kidney) and respiratory organ systems (lungs).

4. **Phthalates** - Used to maintain fragrance and color in products. This batch of chemicals causes hormonal disturbances in women and sterility in men. Worse yet, genital abnormalities have been found in male fetuses after use of these chemicals. In both men and women, it lowers the production of sex hormones. This can lead to various forms of cancer.

5. **Triclosan** - This is a chemical compound that acts as an antibacterial. The use of commercial deodorant or antiperspirant containing triclosan can lead to altering the regulation of hormones. Of course, this is all important for women.

Heard enough? Well, I'm not done quite yet. Some of you are getting your minds going as two alternatives you can choose besides the poisonous staple you've been using thus far. Some of you may be thinking you can go organic, while others of you may be thinking of how you can concoct some sort of special brew in your very own kitchen. In any case, I love the proactive thought!

For those of you who are thinking that Tom's of Maine or Nature's Valley Organics is the way to go, they also have some dangerous, skin-penetrating ingredients embedded in them as well. So, what's the solution? After visiting more natural seminars and holistic conventions that I'd like to admit, I found the very best things are the simplest ones. Here is the best alternative you will ever find to a commercial deodorant of any kind...

Lemon Balm. You can buy it or make it, but it only has a few ingredients and it works! Will it last all day? Absolutely. Will it stain my clothes? Not that I have noticed. Does it have any side effects? Yes, it has one. It tends to get rid of migraine headaches! Oh I'm sorry! That's a benefit. *LOL*

That's all! Either find it or make it, but whatever you do, use it. Wouldn't you want someone to ask you, "Hey, who is that smelling lemony fresh?!"

Soap. I know none of you want to leave the house smelling like a duffle bag full of fresh, unwiped ass cracks! That was a little graphic but you get the point. We often utilize the shower or bathtub to wash away the filth from the previous day. This is routine for most people, however, some people don't have this luxury. Others choose to go days without taking a shower or bath... remember those ass cracks I was just talking about? *LOL*

While you are in the process of "denastying" yourself, you are probably using some form of soap or body wash. Once again, you thought these cleaning agents were innocuous and did nothing to your body. However, I have to tell you this is opposite of the truth. Most commercial soaps contain the very same things found in your toothpaste and your deodorant. It's a miracle any of us have survived our morning routine this long!

Just as with the deodorant and toothpaste, I'm going to give you a quick list of risky ingredients found in your bath soaps in an attempt to inform you and give you choice. Here are some of the malignant ingredients found in common hand/body soap provided by http://www.botanicskinessentials.com.

Toxic Soap Ingredients

- 1) Triclosan: Triclosan is a pesticide that has antibacterial properties. ...
- 2) Dioxane: ...
- 3) Sodium laurel sulfate (SLS): ...
- 4) Diethanolamine (or DEA): ...
- 5) Formaldehyde: ...
- 6) Parabens: ...
- 7) Fragrance: ...
- 8) PEG-6:

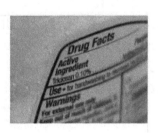

Eight Toxic Soap Ingredients to Avoid - Botanic Skin Essentials
www.botanicskinessentials.com/uncategorized/**toxic-soap-ingredients/**

Do any of these look familiar to you? If they do, you might have seen them in the previous condiments I've already commented on above. Formaldehyde?! Don't they put that in dead people? Never mind the fact that it's also found in most vaccines disseminated today. I won't go into a lengthy discussion on the components of soap. Just know that they are hazardous to your health and you should avoid them at any cost.

Just like with the deodorant and toothpaste, I do have a solution for this one as well. I only use vegan soap in my house. In public, I am subject to whatever the restaurant owners have purchased for me to douse my hands with. However, at home, I'm the boss! Nothing that enters the doors of my home has not been scrutinized down to the very fine print on the label! In fact, I started to make my own soap, when I discovered one of my family members already does the same thing. So I decided to call her up and bought a whole bunch of her soaps.

If you would like to do the same and buy the exact same soap I'm using on a daily basis, you can contact Zelphia on Facebook to buy your own supply. Her website is http://HealthWealthHerbals.com. I kid you not, I have 30 bars of her soap in my bathroom at this very moment! I know that might be a bit of overkill but it's better to be safe than sorry. My skin stays soft and moisturized most of the day, and the best part is...no harmful chemicals! Here's a pic of her website...

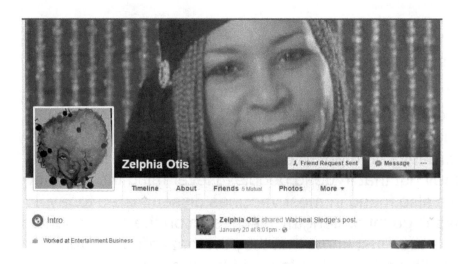

That's all I have for this chapter. Hopefully, you picked up some important information that will help you get rid of any condition or disease that you're dealing with by elimination of these unsafe products. I don't claim to have all the answers, but the ones I do have, work extraordinarily well!

Coming up is the last chapter in this section.

Section Three

Do You Suffer From Any Of These?

Secret #15: Yellow Skin Tone?

It's Friday night, you're looking good, and you're almost done with the finishing touches on your spectacular outfit for the evening. You almost feel invincible getting ready for this amazing night. Your hair came out perfect, your outfit cost you two weeks salary, but who cares, you look like a million bucks! Your friends come by and scoop you up so you all can head to the club in style. You hop into your best friend's new ride... perfect for this unforgettable evening. Off to the club. You all arrive in style in the new Tesla Model S in front of the club and the line is around the building!

You step out of the back passenger door like a boss! There is nothing that can stop you from enjoying this night. You walk into the packed club with the lights dancing off everybody's freshly done hair, their newly purchased outfits, and superbly lotioned skin. You need a drink to loosen up...this is intense! You just got here, and this is the most fun you've had in six months. After you take your tequila shot, it's time to hit the dance floor. You see a group of strangers of the opposite sex on the floor, you approach, then just jump in the middle of them and start going nuts! This is what life should be like. After 6 hours in the club and about 11 drinks, you realize that you are stone-cold wasted!

Your friends take off with their one night stands, so you summon an Uber to chauffeur you home in the wee hours of the morning. You miraculously find the keyhole to open your apartment door, you don't even lock the door behind you, and you pass out obliviously until later that afternoon. Twelve hours later, you wake up with a splitting headache, a severely wrinkled outfit, and an appetite big enough to eat a 10-stack of Cracker Barrel pancakes! When you go to the restroom to look at yourself in the mirror, you look like hell! The fact is, your body took a beating on this epic evening. On the contrary, you actually had a buddy to take that hit for you... that buddy is your LIVER!

The Liver. Our liver is the most regenerative and hard-working organ we have. If I were two cut off a lobe of your liver, it would grow back within a matter of months like a snake's tail! When I say regenerative, I mean it! To put into perspective how important your liver is, let me put this another way. If you were to get into a horrible car accident that mangled your body and vital organs, you could actually live with no brain function at all. However, if you lost your liver during the accident, your body would fail almost immediately!

Having said that, our livers perform over 500 function within the body. It's pretty awesome to know we have an all-in-one organ capable of keeping us alive in the event of emergencies. Let me show you a small fraction of what your liver can do…

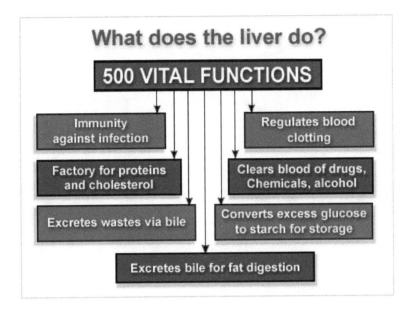

(Graphic was created and modified by Human Health Link, Inc.)

These seem like some very important functions, if I do say so myself. All of which seem to be keeping you alive at this very moment. Us human beings are more geared towards visual stimulation rather than verbal. So I'm going to show you a chart that actually shows you how important your liver is and why it's important to take care of it, no matter what. The chart below shows how our liver cleanses the toxins coming in from many different avenues outside our body. Get this, those same poisons filtered by your liver, leave through the very same pathways they came in.

The Process of Detoxification and Elimination

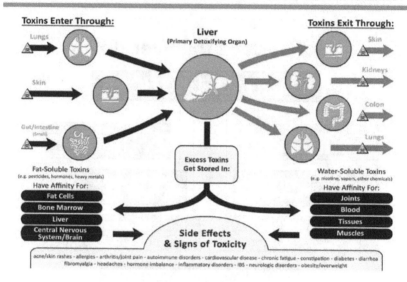

(Graphic was created and modified by Human Health Link, Inc.)

In case you can't read the 'side effects and signs of toxicity' at the bottom of this graphic, they read as follows: acne, skin rashes, allergies, arthritis pain, autoimmune disorders, cardiovascular disease, chronic fatigue, constipation, diabetes, diarrhea, fibromyalgia, headaches, hormone imbalance, inflammatory disorders, IBS, neurologic disorders, and obesity/weight gain. It sounds to me like if your liver is messed up, so are you!

Let's dig a little deeper on this subject. I've read a lot of medical books and articles describing the functions of the liver. There seems to be a common theme with the level of toxicity and liver function. Here's the simple truth of taking care of your liver and how it will affect your health. The magic number is 33%. What does that number mean? The simplest way I can describe it is when your liver hits 33% in functionality, all hell breaks loose!

You see, you can be at 100%, 70%, or even 50% function and still have hardly any diseases, conditions, or syndromes occurring in your body at any given time. Be that as it may, as soon as you hit the 33% number, you're visits to the doctor will surely begin.

For some of us, going to the doctor has become a strong habit. If you really think about it, sick people go to the hospital. If you are well, there is really no need to visit a hospital, not even for a check-up! Admit it to yourself... you only go to the doctor because other people around you are doing the same thing. Every time something goes wrong, don't you automatically think you should go see your family physician? Tell the truth! I'll put myself in your shoes, I've been conditioned just like you, and years before I wrote this book, I visited the doctor's office for every single thing that went wrong with my body. That is very hard to admit, being that I'm telling you not to do so now.

What I'm telling you is HEALTH HAPPENS AT HOME! Whatever chronic condition you have, you can diagnose, treat, and cure in your personal, home kitchen. Let's not overlook the obvious, If you have an acute injury that requires immediate attention, you should go to the emergency room of a hospital. In fact, that is the only room in the hospital I recommend you visit during your lifetime. Notwithstanding, I know some of you are stubborn to a fault. You won't give up your addiction to your drugs or your doctor, no matter what I say! Hey, I'm not here to try to tell you how to run your life. I'm only presenting facts so that you can make an informed decision. Moving on.

Alcohol and Your Liver. Our liver stores toxins within its hepatic cells from the time we were born! This means our liver never gets a break. Those poisons accumulate over the years causing the liver to slowdown in its function. One of the ways to make sure these poisoned accumulate quicker is by ingesting alcohol. I know some of you really don't want to hear that! Nonetheless, you have to if you really want to change your health and well-being. Alcohol is a very good way to get to that 33% number really fast!

Cirrhosis is long-term damage to the liver. One of the biggest cues you are experiencing late-stage damage in your liver is the color of your skin. Yellowing of the skin (jaundice) is caused by a buildup of a by-product from your red blood cells called bilirubin. Why is this building up in your skin? The yellow color in our skin usually indicates advanced liver disease. This means the liver is hardly working, if at all. The liver can no longer store toxins, therefore, the waste products have to be stored elsewhere. The farthest place away from your healthy blood supply is your skin tissue.

Healthy   Cirrhosis

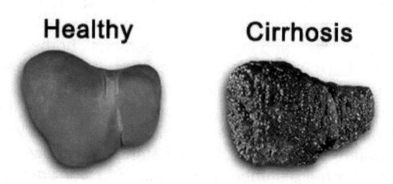

Think about this for just a second, you eat foods laced with chemicals, additives, and preservatives. Some of you smoke cigarettes packed with tar and nicotine.

Others of you take a toke of the marijuana or hookah in an attempt to make your life more enjoyable (I might have to agree with this one...*LOL*). Yet and still, a small percentage of you indulge in hardcore drugs like cocaine, heroin, or meth. Now, top this off with alcohol and you just created a super highway to 33%!

When the liver is bombarded with numerous toxins over a long period of time, the function of the liver will decrease inevitably. Once the function of the liver gets to a point where toxins are no longer allowed into the liver, our blood will start searching for other pathways to funnel the poisons to, in an attempt to keep it out of the blood (see "Cirrhosis" above).

For instance, taking prescription or over-the-counter medications may relieve your symptoms temporarily. Acknowledging this, the byproducts are left for your body to dispose of. Because our bodies don't have an effective way of disposing of these offshoots, they are simply stored in our tissues. Some of the main places these poisons end up are our joints, our cartilage, and the soft tissues of our vital organs (like the liver). Have you ever heard of an autoimmune disease? It's a rather common diagnosis these days.

Is there really such a thing as an autoimmune disease? No! I have yet to come across a traditional medical book that says an autoimmune disease is caused by poisons accumulating in our body tissues. They all say our body is *mistakenly* attacking itself. This nonchalant attitude about how are body works has nothing to do with science or study. So let me ask you this, if our bodies are making mistakes and doctors don't know what's causing them, then how are they prescribing medication for something they don't understand?

An autoimmune disease is the act of our white blood cells (leukocytes) attacking our own body tissues. Our body is supremely intelligent and requires no outside help in order to repair itself, with the exception of acute, deep injuries from the outside. In the case of autoimmune diseases, our leukocytes are actively searching to kill invaders all day, every day, and in real-time. If our leukocytes appear to be attacking our own body tissue, it's only because there are antigens present in the tissue that need to be disposed of.

Here's the good news in all of this...I've found the human body has a 10 to 1 recovery ratio when it comes to most aspects of healing. Meaning if you abused your body by drinking alcohol for 10 years, all you have to do is take care of it for one year, and it rebounds all the way back to normal! This is true for the liver as well.

Getting Your Liver Back. We can go hard or we can go soft, but in any case, we're going! I didn't mean to sound like one of your average, run-of-the-mill action stars in a cheesy movie. I only meant to tell you there are two ways to cleanse your liver to bring it back to optimum, and get back above that 33% and beyond.

1. Method #1 (Soft Method): We perform a whole body cleanse, and I don't mean a colonic. When doing the whole body cleanse, I recommend the Gaia Supreme Cleanse. Most colonics only flush the colon. We want a more effective, deep cleanse of our tissues. Thus, we are going to clean the colon, tissues, and liver. The

instructions are pretty clear for this thorough, 14-day cleanse. The instructions go over what to eat, and more importantly, what not to eat. This method will take about two weeks and is considered the "slow" method of cleansing the liver.

2. Method #2 (Hard Method): If you are not concerned with anything else and only want to clean the liver, I suggest the coffee enema. "What?! You want me to shoot coffee up my butt?!" Yup! Didn't you know, the best part of waking up, is Folgers in your butt! *LMAO*

Coffee enemas utilize the hepatic portal vein in order to route the coffee to the liver. The reason we use coffee is because it's a stimulant. This will agitate the tissues of the liver so that it will release all of the toxins stored in the hepatic cells. This method alone could jump your liver function back up to 70% easily! Numerous coffee enemas could get you back to 100% in just months. I have a video on how to properly do a coffee enema.

I always warn about temperature when doing them. **Never attempt to do a coffee enema with hot coffee!** You should always check temperature (it should be slightly above room temperature) before ever inserting the anal tube. In addition, make sure you emptied your bowels before doing a coffee enema. We want to minimize pushback during the holding of the coffee. **(Coffee enema video: https://www.youtube.com/watch?v=-iiHDCOVv_Y)**

I have just one more graphic to show you detailing what the liver does for us before I leave this chapter. Take a look at the graphic below. It's pretty amazing what your liver can do when it's healthy. Having said that, it's pretty amazing how fast your health can decline if your liver is not functioning correctly.

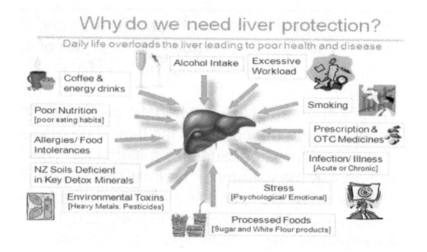

(Graphic was created and modified by Human Health Link, Inc.)

I hope I provided enough value to persuade you to take care of your liver, and maybe even invigorate it. The methods I've outlined in this chapter are not difficult to complete in the least. Take your time, do your own research, and find out what works best for your body. My way is not always the best way, it's just the best way for me!

That ends this section and this chapter. I'll be taking you into a new section where we'll talk about some of the interests involved in keeping your health at a minimum and profits at a maximum. It's not easy to hear, but it's ultimately necessary to provide an understanding of why this is happening to us. If this bothers you, so what! My mission is not to make everyone happy. My goal in writing this book is to disseminate the best information possible, so you can make an educated choice in the healthcare decisions you make every day!

Section Four

Do You Suffer From Any Of These?

Secret #16: Profit Above All...F*** Your Health!

Let me start by saying I believe doctors are good people, I believe they go to church, I believe they really want to help, but they cannot have your best interest at heart! How can I make such a strong statement? Well, if you knew the history of how Western medicine came to power, you wouldn't have any doubts about what I'm saying at all. Maybe you've noticed you are treated more like a lead in a hospital instead of a patient. You're treated more like a number rather than a person. Often times, the doctor walks into the room and doesn't even look your way until it's time for you to pay. Does that sound like personal health care to you? HELL NO!

You might have doubts about what I'm saying or you may not believe me at all. Trust me, I understand. You like your doctor, you like going to their office, and you appreciate the good job they do when they see you.

Nonetheless, all doctors are trained in the same methods of cut, burn, and poison! Translation... surgery, radiation, and pharmaceutical drugs.

Your doctor is nothing but part of a network meant to disseminate authoritarian information, making you the hapless victim that follows orders (doctor's orders). It really doesn't matter if your doctor is nice or arrogant, God-fearing or Atheist, focused or indifferent. The fact is, most information you receive from a physician will get you killed! Let me reintroduce some information you may not have heard of or might have forgotten...

Doctors are not pharmacists! Most of the time, doctors are giving you samples of drugs which have no safety testing, and even worse, unknown side effects that have not been discovered yet. From personal experience, I can tell you the most a doctor knows about the pharmaceutical poison he's doling out to you is what the sales rep. told him when she dropped off the samples! Does that make you feel good about taking drugs from your "doc"? You may as well walk up to a homeless man and ask him for a couple hits of his personal stash. It's the same thing! Neither one knows what the hell they're giving you.

With that said, let me bestow upon you some history of how this demonic version of Western medicine came to be in America. Here are some facts you can freely look up on your own, should you choose to. I found this information quite disturbing but it's validated by more than one source. I hope you find this information interesting and hope it lights a fire under your ass to start taking care of your body AT HOME...and not at a damned hospital!

1910: John D. Rockefeller sends Abraham Flexner to Congress to begin reform of the medical industry by attempting to outlaw anything outside the scope of surgery, radiation, and patentable drugs.

1911: The United States Supreme Court finds John D. Rockefeller guilty of corruption, racketeering, and illegal business practices. Soon after, the Rockefeller Standard Oil Trust was sentenced to be dismantled. It appears Rockefeller is above the decision of the Supreme Court and not concerned at all about this ruling.

1913: The heat is still on Rockefeller. In order to disperse some of this negative attention, he creates the Rockefeller Foundation. He funneled money from his illegal business activities into his not-for-profit. His foundation is used to fund medical schools and hospitals under the auspices of philanthropy. This influence gives Rockefeller control over the doctors decisions and enables him to push pharmaceutical, patentable drugs onto the market at an alarming rate. This was also the time when scientists started to discover that vitamins and minerals could stop, and even reverse disease! This was an amazing breakthrough, however, it was not good for Rockefeller business. Thus, he went to the United Nations in order to get less civilized countries to ban vitamins and minerals as a way to treat disease.

1918: The public starts to realize the importance of vitamins and minerals, which severely halts the progression of pharmaceutical drugs. Not one to let competition reign in a free market, Rockefeller uses the Spanish flu epidemic along with public media (a company he owned already) to block out every form of medicine that was not pharmaceutical drugs. Within the span of 15 years, medical schools, hospitals, and the American Medical Association all became Rockefeller's peons! Rockefeller would continue to use his foundation to push his agenda overseas...and succeeded.

1925: Competition arises in Germany for Global control of the pharmaceutical drug market. It seems Rockefeller's involvement overseas has made him some enemies. The German cartel known as I.G. Farben uses the same method Rockefeller used to divide up the United States, only they do this globally. To these Titans of corruption, the world is ripe for the picking.

1929: Both the Rockefeller Foundation and I.G. Farben decided to divide the globe into "interest zones" (sale territories).

1932-1933: I.G. Farben is not happy with the arrangement with the Rockefeller Foundation. They decide to vault their position ahead by jumping into the political game. They back a German dictator (Hitler) to overthrow the present leadership in exchange for a favor. They want to start a war to promote chaos, so they may profit from the inevitable fallout health-wise. They are successful with their coup. This was the beginning of World War II!

In every country Hitler's Wehrmacht (defense force) invaded, their mission was to take out the pharmaceutical, chemical, and petrochemical institutions, which would all be replaced with I.G. Farben pharmaceuticals.

1942-1945: In order to solidify its global, pharmaceutical position, I.G. Farben tests their pharmaceuticals on concentration camp inmates in Auschwitz, Dachau. The payments used to conduct these inhumane experiments came directly from the bank accounts of Bayer, BASF, and Hoechst, going directly to the bank of the concentration camps.

1945: The big plan does not pay off! I.G. Farben backs the wrong side of the war and losses World War II. This enables a takeover of I.G. Farben by the Rockefeller Foundation, JPMorgan, and The Rothschilds.

1947: In the Nuremberg war crimes tribunal, members of the involved companies were tried for crimes against humanity. However, the executives of I.G. Farben (the ones who actually started the wars and inhumane experiments) got the mildest of sentences.

In 1944, Nelson Rockefeller had already been made part of the executive branch of the United States government. This would solidify John Rockefeller's hold on corruption and ensure that it would continue. In fact, the culprits who ended nearly 60 million lives during the Holocaust would not only escape hanging, but would be completely exonerated. As you will see, they were needed later.

1949: The Federal Republic of Germany was founded. This would serve as a transatlantic outpost for the interests of the Rockefellers. Within only a few years, the managers of I.G. Farben were released from jail and reinstated to their previous positions has heads of the Rockefeller Trust. One of the executive managers, Fritz Ter Meer, was again chairman of the largest

German multi-national pharmaceutical company, Bayer by 1963!

1945-1949: The Rockefeller Brothers founded the United Nations. This was a clever ploy to protect their interests globally, which has more authority than localized government. The United Nations is composed of nearly 200 countries, however, only three countries really have any power. The others are merely background scenery for the US and its drug pushing allies. The World Health Organization and the World Trade Organization are nothing but political arms of the drug & pharmaceutical company's interests.

1963: The Rockefellers addiction to Greed has no bounds. They launched a 40-year campaign to outlaw all natural means of medicine. That includes vitamins and minerals, along with any non-patentable health alternative. The Rockefellers and their business partners see this form of bullying as necessary for complete control of the planet! This corrupt consortium knows the eradication of disease cannot be the goal, thus, pharmaceutical drugs are never meant to heal or cure any disease.

This begins the era of allopathic medicine. Only treating the symptoms ensures the patient will never get well and will therefore, be obligated to take medications for the rest of their lives!

Linus Pauling and other brave scientist deserve immense credit for their efforts in keeping the door open for Americans to know exactly what they're putting into their bodies. Mr. Pauling is directly responsible for spreading the scientific word of vitamins and minerals as necessary for prolonged health. Linus also deserves credit for bringing up the incredible work of Dr. Rath. Dr. Rath conducted experiments and found that nutrients missing from the heart we're almost solely responsible for heart disease.

1990-1992: These years signify the beginning of the end of pharmaceutical reign over our lives. Dr. Rath, with co-author Linus Pauling, published a series a scientific papers proving micronutrient deficiency was the main cause of most disease! These diseases include heart attacks, high blood pressure, diabetes, circulatory problems, cancer and even immune deficiency diseases, including AIDS.

By tracing the information sources back to their origin, Dr. Rath could conclude only one thing, the information was being hidden for the diabolical interests of pharmaceutical drug companies.

~ [Dr. Rath Health Foundation, The History of the Pharma-Cartel. http://www4.dr-rath-foundation.org/THE_FOUNDATION/history_of_the_pharma_cartel.html]

Just to expound on that last point a little bit further, it is illegal for a doctor to inform you of the health benefits of a cranberry today! It seems that more and more doctors are getting tired of watching their patients reappear sicker and sicker, and some even encountering early death. There are fine lines overlaid on our corrupt medical profession. A physician can tell a patient to improve their diet or even suggest some food they can eat, but they cannot inform the patient of the benefits of each food. What?! Are you as fed up as I am?!

I do apologize for the length of this history lesson, however, some of you will never believe the kind of evil you are being controlled by. My job is to inform you to provide CHOICE and not make you one of the inmates in this American concentration camp!

BONUS: I'm Just Doing My Job!

This very phrase is the reason Americans cannot and will not come together in the future for their own common interest! I mean this, so listen carefully, as you may have done this to someone in your life and not even realized it.

Have you ever asked a police officer to forgive your ticket? Of course you have, none of us want to take a ticket. Think about the consequences of him giving you your ticket, your insurance may go up, you have to pay a ticket that could be anywhere from $75 to $400, or you may even have to show up in court! The officer in front of you knows full well the consequences of giving you this ticket. Nonetheless in a robotic voice he will tell you, "I'm just doing my job", then he gives you the ticket anyway! The one thing that pisses me off the most about this: Humans are being trained to become robots!

In some cases as simple as this, the attending officer could be f***ing up your life! Does anyone care? Does he care? Nope! He's just doing his job. The sad thing is, we've all done this to other people at some time or another in our lives. Unity cannot occur while social norms like this exist. I'm guilty of this very same phrase myself.

I'll supply you with a personal example. One of my students missed turning in a homework assignment that had a pretty heavy effect on their final average. I don't allow students to turn in late homework if the class is closed, and in this case, the class was already over. To be honest, I could have taken the students homework, put it into the system, and no one would have known the difference. Unfortunately, I didn't do that. I stuck to the school policy and refuse to take the paper from the student. The student, coincidentally, failed the class because they missed this one assignment. I guess you could say, I was just doing my job. Going forward, I can't help but think I made another human being's life worse. That's a hard thing to try to deal with as an instructor but it happens more often than you'd think.

Could the student have come back to me and got me to change my mind? Probably, I'm pretty flexible when it comes to situations like this. Did the student come back and ask me a second time? No. I have to tell you, sometimes I wish they would come back and fight for what they believe is important. To me, rules are guidelines that can be deviated from when a human being needs help from another human being. Rules and regulations should not be hard and fast constraints we have to live by, no matter what, under the guise of "doing our job"!

Here's where you come in. I want you to go back to your doctor a second time and ask for more information. I want you to ask more questions, be more aggressive, and demand your health be taken seriously! Second opinion, third opinion, maybe even a fourth opinion may be necessary, but I want you to do it! Your health is important! If you are going to leave your well-being to the control of a corrupt, unscrupulous, and uncaring group of evil executives, then you will get what you ask for.

BONUS #2: I Didn't Go To School For Nothing!

There is one part of this corrupt system I believe is not your physician's fault. Retail pharmaceutical drug companies fund medical schools, hospitals, and the American Medical Association. These institutions have all become pawns in a business plan to bankrupt the health of American citizens. Due to the influence of "Big Pharma", doctors feel obligated to peddle patented drugs as restitution for drug companies helping them get through medical school.

There is one more string attached to the arms of these medical marionettes, they have huge tuition bills! I believe the sole reason for a physician's education being so high is to indenture them. This creates an incentive for the doctor to push for higher priced procedures that will bring him a higher return to help pay back these shoulder-crushing student loans. Now let's add malpractice insurance, taxes, alimony, and other medical expenses used to keep his medical office open. All these charges, fees, and payments on top of those student loans, almost puts a gun to the doctors he head to charge you for unnecessary services to recoup his investment on his education!

You have to understand, when the motive is money, your health has to come second, by definition! The main goal of any *business* is to make money. If we turn hospitals into businesses, our health will always be a distant second to the bottom line. The ability to pay should never be a consideration in a health care system, especially in a system considered one of the richest in the world.

That's going to conclude this chapter and I hope you didn't feel my disdain too much for the unethical treatment of my fellow human beings. Buck up! All of the above might sound absolutely terrible. So I'm going to provide you with some solutions in the next chapter to help you circumvent this exploitive health care system.

Section Four

Do You Suffer From Any Of These?

Secret #17: Wallets Unite!

So far I have brought you a nice positive-negative mix of medical information. It is my hope you've enjoyed what you've read so far. Now it is time to cement an idea in your mind. Hollywood might call this 'Inception'! This is not my idea, this is your idea, which you have very deep in your mind but never had the courage to say out loud in the presence of your doctor. It's an idea that lingers...almost tapping at the back of your brain. It's an idea so primitive, so simple, so persistent, yet you fail to listen to the tiny voice guiding you. What am I talking about? The simplest words none of us like to whisper to ourselves...

IS THIS RIGHT???

For two weeks you've been having rapid heartbeat, heart palpitations, migraine headaches and abdominal pain. After you can't take it anymore, off to the doctor you go. He runs 500 tests that all come back normal. They tell you, "Take this (medicine) and see if anything changes". How can your practitioner prescribe medication for something when all your tests acknowledge nothing exists?! You should be thinking to yourself, "Is this right?"

You get a Papanicolaou (pap smear) done, only to discover you have fibroids and worse yet, polycystic ovarian syndrome (PCOS). At present, you are only 20 years old, but the OB GYN "strongly recommends" you have a complete hysterectomy. After this rather harsh diagnosis, you might be thinking to yourself, "Wouldn't that completely shut down my female hormone production and prevent me from ever having kids naturally? Is this right?"

A strange mole, you've never seen before, seems to be growing on the backside of your left shoulder. It makes you nervous, so you head to the dermatologist's office. Upon inspection, they recommend a biopsy. Two weeks later, the test shows positive for cancer cells. Your skin doctor recommends you have the lesion excised. If they find further cancer cells, they will cut out even more flesh, and this process will continue until the cancer is gone. The "doc" utters firmly, "Fair warning! This process may take us down to the bone!" (This does happen, quite often). One more time, "There has to be a better way! Is this right?"

The above examples are all too common in our Western medical system. You will be treated for symptoms not causes. You will be prescribed medications not minerals. You will be guided to surgeries and not home solutions! A state of pure rage overtakes me every time I hear a student, a friend, or family member tell me about their vicious run-ins with these money-hungry slaughterhouses! Now we know the history of the problems and we know the problems are real. So what's the solution to all of this?

Well, It's not what most medical reform specialist are saying on television! They believed that we need critical reform. Others believe we need a comprehensive overhaul of the entire system. I believe a none of this will lead to the solution you or I want. Allow me to elaborate, whether we have an overtly corrupt system or a slightly corrupt system, there are two things common in both...CORRUPTION!

Trying to change a unethical system is an exercise in futility. The accomplishments of a corrupt system are not built on merit, they are built on profit! What's right often comes last to the bottom line. This American dictatorship disguised as a republic will protect its interests, no matter what. We have police trained to be robots and follow orders at any given moment. We also have lobbyists as a native part of government, which means corruption is, literally, built into the system! If you've got the money, you've got the vote!

On the opposite foot, if you sell healthy milk, vitamins, and minerals to the public, the FDA will come and shut you down for spreading good health throughout America! If you speak out about vaccines and do your own clinical trials to prove MMR, in fact, causes autism, you will end up face-down in a river! Ask Dr. Jeffrey Bradstreet. Here's the worst part, if you tell the average American they could cure their cancer within six months without ever visiting a hospital, they wouldn't believe you. When "the system" has your mind, there is no hope for you!

Please! There has to be a solution to all of this? Of course there is, and it's even more elementary than you thought possible. This will not be done by comprehensive health care reform, nor will it be accomplished by a complete system overhaul. Both the cause and the solution to this problem are the same thing...MONEY!

One thing I've noticed throughout history in America is money does not stop! No matter what the crisis, the money must keep flowing in order for America to remain great. That being the case, corruption has actually played a huge part in keeping our economy going. Nonetheless, we cannot have corruption enter the healthcare field, as it eliminates too many lives. Wholeheartedly, I know money is the answer.

The entire system we refer to as Western Medical Care is based on the American citizen paying premiums to an insurance company. The advent of insurance to pay for health care costs was one of the worst inventions ever brought upon civilized society. Because insurance companies can pay hospitals in large lump sums, this enables hospitals and surgery centers to charge exorbitant fees for their services. Even better, Joe citizen only has to pay a small premium over time without ever having to come out of pocket for the entire cost. Needless to say, this breeds corruption and dependency.

The answer is simple: KEEP YOUR MONEY IN YOUR F***ING POCKET! I'm not saying this to be mean or vulgar, I'm saying it because it's true. Let's assess, no doctor's visit means no doctor fee, no surgical operation means no surgical fee, and no chemotherapy means you can eliminate 10 rounds of "chemo" at $7,000 apiece! Most people are so reliant on this present system, if I advised them to stop paying insurance premiums, they would become violent towards me!

It's beyond me how we have become so dependent on the system. When companies lose money (and that's all hospitals are), policies tend to change...real quick! Think about this a little bit more deeply, when citizens made runs on the bank in times of depression, the banks quickly closed their doors to stem the flow of money out there doors. Money they probably didn't have! In the case of Bernie Madoff, he ran the largest Ponzi scheme in American financial history! The only reason the roof came down is because investors demanded their money back and Bernie was wasn't able to deliver.

It seems when the American public makes demands in staggering numbers, they can stop any corrupt institution from prospering. This includes the dubious Western medical system! Stop taking medications that take decades off your life. Stop going to institutions that treat you as a number on the sheet instead of a real human being. Lastly, stop paying your money to a system that is laughing behind your back all the way to the bank as you become further and further raped by debt!

Now that I have had my peace, are you ready for the last chapter? I'll give you some final takeaways and things you can use right now to boost your health for the long term. Flip the page, I'll see you there.

Section Four

Do You Suffer From Any Of These?

Secret #18: Your Kitchen vs. Your Hospital Room

What you do for yourself at home is more powerful than any treatment that could come out of any hospital! This may be hard to believe for some of you, especially the ones of you who visit hospitals on a regular basis. It might be an impossible notion to believe we can achieve perfect health without MRIs, blood glucose tests, multiple diagnoses, and fancy, heavily equipped medical buildings. If you feel this way, hopefully some of the information I've provided in this book has, at least, shed some light on your perspective. For those of you who passionately believe we can do extraordinary things at home, read on!

The truth *is* I haven't gone to see a doctor in over 12 years! This may seem unfathomable for some of you. I don't need constant checkups to make sure my health is okay. I don't need numerous x-rays to show me that my bones are healthy. I don't need an EEG to tell me if my brain is functioning properly. How can I go all these years without having any tests of any kind and still be walking around healthy as a horse?! The answer: I pay attention to how I feel.

If you can't do this yet, don't worry. It took me a long time to trust my body and my feelings, and it will take a bit of time for you. Most of us don't have the balls to stand up to our doctors and tell them what we really want from our medical treatment. Some of you are too afraid to tell your doctor you don't want to take his advice! Let me get this straight, you're going to sit there and let the doctor dictate how you should live the rest of your life, after his extremely thorough 10-minute assessment?! You've known your body for 29 years, and all of a sudden he's an expert on your entire life in 10 minutes? Get f***ing serious!

The healthiest people on this planet seldom visit the doctor. If you don't believe me, I'll wait just a minute while you do a Google search to find out what are some of the most successful attributes of a person living to 100, go ahead I'll wait.

These miraculous people who live to 100 years old are call centenarians. Living a century of life has to be an extremely fulfilling accomplishment, especially if you've lived this life to the fullest! At this present moment, I don't believe most Americans will ever make it anywhere near this magical number. I'm not saying this because I don't want it to happen, I'm saying this because it's almost an impossibility at present.

In 2015 and 2016, we had the first decline in American age longevity since 1993. These are not promising numbers, as technology has improved greatly in the medical field. However, our health is only getting worse. That's an amazing conundrum that we can't help but think about.

Take time to think about this, we have the most accomplished medical schools in the world, spend at least 10X more than any other country per capita on healthcare, and we rank 27th in the world in overall health. The United States is highest among infant mortality rates, sickness and disease, and lowest in satisfaction with our healthcare system. Something's wrong! When I experience problems with my health, this sounds like the last place I would visit.

Let me propose an alternative. The next time something goes wrong with your body, in lieu of performing your morning ritual of getting dressed, loading yourself into your car, and driving across town to your nearest disease management facility, I'd like you to take the 22-step journey to your kitchen instead.

Most bodily problems arise from one of two things, toxicity or deficiency. If the body is toxic (poisoned), then it's very easy for diseases to proliferate throughout our bodies. However, if our bodies are more on the basic side of the pH scale, it's nearly impossible for any disease to take hold and spread. When we refer to deficiency, we mean the body is lacking in vital micronutrients necessary for our survival.

Just a reminder, our food supply is not sufficient for acquiring all the micronutrients we need on a daily basis. Our daily values have slowly gone down as our diet has become consistent with "foodstuffs" (an FDA term) instead of real food. Supplementation is necessary in the modern era, as made evident by Dr. Rath.

Your Hospital Room. I cringe at the thought, but some of you find this room in your local hospital rather soothing. The subtle smell of industrial aprons, the unmistakable scent of death, and the twerking of Jell-O on your plastic, manila meal tray. Doesn't it just make you want to take a vacation there? No!

Never mind that your nurse has an attitude, no one has come to see you in 8 months, and your health keeps declining despite 24-hour health monitoring. Let's add the fact that you can't walk on your own, additional medications are added to your chart every month, and the only time you see your family is in pictures. Are you depressed yet, because I sure am!

I can't believe some of my family members would prefer to go through this subtle form of hell at the suggestion of their physician! When you read it on paper, doesn't it sound a little bit more sinister? Doesn't it make you wonder if human beings should ever have to go through this? Is this right?

EEGs, EKGs, MRIs, CTs, HTCs, HBGs, PSAs...WTF! Do you even know what any of this s*** means? Do you even ask when these anonymous letters show up on your chart? I know, I know. Some of you don't care as long as they make you feel better, right? I know pain is powerful and emotional, therefore, the average person will accept anything (even at the risk of their health) to get rid of it! After all, that's one of our deepest psychological presets...the avoidance of pain.

This avoidance of pain is enough to make you suffer through all of the events I've mentioned above.

Your Kitchen. There might be grease stains on your microwave, leftover bacon on your stove, and dishwashing liquid caked on the sink, but from now on, this is going to be your "clinic"! Your kitchen is no longer the place where you open your fast food bags, unload your sugary cereals, or store your boots for the winter (for those of you in New York). *Haha*

We are now going to refer to this as your "culinary pharmacy". Oh, you don't believe natural food, along with vitamins and minerals can help you get rid of common illnesses? I would disagree! As a matter of fact, let me give you just five common conditions that may be quite severe, and the nutritional equivalents how to correct them.

Condition	Traditional Treatment	"Wholistic" Treatment
Cold	Cough Syrup, Nasal Decongestant	Carrot, Pineapple, Ginger, Garlic
Memory Loss	Cholinesterase Inhibitors	Pomegranate, Beets, Grapes (Red)
High Blood Pressure	Diuretics, Beta-blockers, Ace-inhibitors, Blood Vessel Dilators	Beets, Apple, Celery Cucumber, Ginger

Asthma	Inhaler, Nebulizer	Carrot, Spinach, Apple, Garlic, Lemon
Depression	SSRIs	Carrot, Apple, Spinach, Beets

Check the back of this book for even more conditions and natural food remedies!

Now all you have to do is pick up a NutriBullet, NutriNinja, or any other fancy blender on the market today that will liquefy all these beautiful foods. Those of you who are into spending 30 minutes to clean a juicer after you're done with it, I'd recommend a regular juicer (Jack Lalane Juice Machine) instead of the NutriBullet. Some swear that a juicer will preserve more nutrients in the fruits and vegetables. I found through tragic personal experience, using a traditional juicer instead of a power blender (like the NutriBullet) will manifest staggering grocery bills!

Here's an example, it takes 15 carrots to make one glass of carrot juice with a traditional juicer. It only takes three carrots and some filtered water to make one glass of carrot juice with a NutriBullet. You choose which one works best for you, I'm just telling you what I've done in my own kitchen.

I hope you noticed by now, I am not an advocate of perfection or being pure. Some believe you should rid your body of every single antigen and microorganism. That is an impossibility! On top of that, you have an immune system for a reason. If you eat pure all the time and never encounter external antigens, your white blood cells won't know how to fight anything once it does attack your body.

As with anything in our bodies, if you don't use it, you lose it! If you have cells that are supposed to attack invaders within our blood, how effective do you think they'll be if they've never fought a battle before? It is my conclusion from going through this life that our human bodies are made stronger by adversity! Being exposed to microorganisms is what builds a strong immune system. Ever seen 'War of the Worlds'?

Don't believe me? Ask anyone with leukemia if they would rather have a strong immune system to fight off the invaders attacking them on a daily basis, ultimately ending their life! If you know nothing about leukemia, it's called a cancer of the blood. However, it acts like anything but. With most forms of leukemia, the body is unable to produce effective white blood cells to fight off foreign antigens. This often results in the death of the patient. Had the body been allowed to adapt at earlier stages, the white blood cells could strengthen their defense power and eradicated invading diseases.

What about small children who have leukemia? They "inherited" this awful disease from their parents. When I say inherit, I don't mean they got it genetically. It's more serious than that. In most cases, the parents developed compromised blood quality via very poor eating habits, exposure to daily toxins, breathing in pollutants, and being injected with poisons on a regular basis. The latest studies show most infants born this century have, on average, 232 chemicals and pollutants in their umbilical cord without having lived a day on this planet!

You see, the more we go along with this suicidal convention, our children's life spans are cut shorter and shorter! I don't believe this has to be the case. I BELIEVE in hope beyond hope! It is my mission on this planet to make sure that metabolic disease does not spread to the next generation! You can join me in this unprecedented move, or sit quietly on the sidelines and watch your world be quietly put down.

The Wrap Up. At the beginning of this book, I gave you a quote by Hippocrates. It stated, "Let food be thy medicine, and medicine be thy food". Hippocrates lived from 460 BC to 370 BC. This health-conscious philosopher was 90 years old when he died! In those days, this was considered impossible. This is what makes his saying above so powerful. He used foods to heal his body, not chemicals, not radiation, and not surgeries.

Yes, you can eliminate stage-four cancers using only food and minerals. Yes, you can get rid of diabetes within 30 days no matter how long you've had it. Yes, you can reverse leukemia and restore your immune system to its normal state. Yes, you can recover from PCOS and begin to plan a family again!

Does this sound impossible? If your answer is yes, then you haven't been listening. You may have to reread this book or do some research of your own to convince yourself that others throughout history have been doing this since the time before Christ.

Dr. Max Gerson was curing late-stage cancers in the 1920's, Dr. Otto Warburg uncovered how to get rid of disease by alkalizing the body in the 1930's, and Dr. Royal Rife put forward the proof that radio frequency waves could reverse disease in the same time period. In the new era, Dr. Stanislaw Burzynski used miraculous particles called antineoplastons to eradicate cancer in difficult cases.

Most people walking around on this planet have no idea who these men are and what they've done for our medical community. They are not just pioneers, they are heroes! They've left behind a legacy of healing and a blueprint to ensure you never have to take illicit drugs to fix your ailing body.

Who would have thought shooting coffee up your butt would cure your cancer and restore your energy levels? Who thought shooting radio waves through your body would restore your health completely? Who thought taking baking soda twice a day for a few months cut completely reverse a stage-four cancer? Did you believe any of these things were possible before you read this book?

Look, this book was never meant to be the end-all-be-all guide to comprehensive human health. On the other hand, this book was created to provide a window to the other side. Before you read this book, you were locked in a room with prescription pharmaceutical drugs, lifelong surgeries, and crippling radiation. I've knocked a hole in the wall so that you can see fruits and vegetables, vitamins and minerals, and life-giving exercise on the other side.

Live food gives you life! A plant-based diet is one of the main staples in keeping any disease from inhabiting your body permanently. Supplementing with the correct vitamins and minerals will ensure your health never declines, and disease will never take over. Exercise will keep your blood moving to supply your vital organs with its necessary nutrients. All of this works together to keep you a healthy human. That makes me happy! Who knows, you might even become one of those centenarians I was talking about!

Feel free to contact me anytime on the media links to follow. I'm always happy to hear stories of success and struggle! It has been my pleasure to write this book for you and my gratitude knows no bounds for you spending your time with me.

Thank you.

THE END

Let me spread some LOVE...

Thank you for reading my book. My hope is you'll read this book more than once. As a matter of fact, I hope you keep reopening it to certain sections until it becomes a raggedy. I want you to leave it out on your counter, so that your friends and family can see what you're doing and maybe they'll follow you on the same path.

I often amaze people with how healthy I am. I don't tell them anything about what I do, the people I help, or how I reversed my own bout with disease. It's almost like they see something in me, something that's glowing, something that extremely vibrant. Some of my students ask me at the end of the sequence, "How do you come in everyday with so much energy?" I always tell them the same thing, "Fruits and vegetables, vitamins and minerals!"

To good health...Cheers!

Case Study (Unedited):

Dear Alvin I started a year ago maybe more not too long in a vegetarian style and I got systematically lower values for cholesterol Last measure was total cholesterol 123 mg\dl and LDL was 63 mg\dl.and protein C reactive high sensibility was 0.56 mg\L.all smaller values and doctor here is not liking that I am independent thinker on my health.But **I prefer to believe in you than on my cardiologist.**

How To Find Me:

Human Health Link (with Alvin Jackson AKA Alvin J.)

Website: http://humanhealthlink.com/ (Contact me here)

Facebook:
https://www.facebook.com/humanhealthlink/

Instagram: humanhealthlink

Twitter: HumanHealthLink

EAT BUTTER
SMOKE MARIJUANA
KILL CANCER and
LIVE TO 100 YEARS OLD!

Alvin Jackson
"The Most Passionate Non-Doctor On The Internet"

HumanHealthLink.com

Copyright © 2017

CPSIA information can be obtained
at www.ICGtesting.com
Printed in the USA
FSHW022005060319
56157FS